T0259388

Falls Prevention

Editor

STEVEN C. CASTLE

CLINICS IN
GERIATRIC MEDICINE

www.geriatric.theclinics.com

May 2019 • Volume 35 • Number 2

ELSEVIER

1600 John F. Kennedy Boulevard • Suite 1800 • Philadelphia, Pennsylvania, 19103-2899

http://www.theclinics.com

CLINICS IN GERIATRIC MEDICINE Volume 35, Number 2
May 2019 ISSN 0749–0690, ISBN-13: 978-0-323-67856-8

Editor: Jessica McCool
Developmental Editor: Laura Fisher

Clinics in Geriatric Medicine (ISSN 0749-0690) is published quarterly by Elsevier Inc., 360 Park Avenue South, New York, NY 10010-1710. Months of issue are February, May, August, and November. Business and Editorial Offices: 1600 John F. Kennedy Blvd., Suite 1800, Philadelphia, PA 191023-2899. Periodicals postage paid at New York, NY, and additional mailing offices. Subscription prices are $286.00 per year (US individuals), $632.00 per year (US institutions), $100.00 per year (US student/resident), $320.00 per year (Canadian individuals), $801.00 per year (Canadian institutions), $195.00 per year (Canadian student/resident), $402.00 per year (international individuals), $801.00 per year (international institutions), and $195.00 per year (international student/resident). Foreign air speed delivery is included in all Clinics subscription prices. All prices are subject to change without notice. POSTMASTER: Send address changes to Clinics in Geriatric Medicine, Elsevier Health Sciences Division, Subscription Customer Service, 3251 Riverport Lane, Maryland Heights, MO 63043. **Telephone: 1-800-654-2452 (U.S. and Canada); 314-447-8871 (outside U.S. and Canada). Fax: 314-447-8029. E-mail:** journalscustomerservice-usa@elsevier. com **(for print support) or** journalsonlinesupport-usa@elsevier.com **(for online support).**

Reprints. For copies of 100 or more, of articles in this publication, please contact the Commercial Reprints Department, Elsevier Inc., 360 Park Avenue South, New York, New York 10010-1710. Tel.: 212-633-3874; Fax: 212-633-3820, E-mail: reprints@elsevier.com.

Clinics in Geriatric Medicine is covered in MEDLINE/PubMed (Index Medicus), EMBASE/Excerpta Medica, Current Contents/Clinical Medicine (CC/CM), and the Cumulative Index to Nursing & Allied Health Literature.

Contributors

EDITOR

STEVEN C. CASTLE, MD
Professor of Geriatric Medicine, UCLA School of Medicine, Clinical Director of Geriatrics, VA Greater Los Angeles, CEO and President, DrBalance, Inc, Certified FallProof! Instructor, California State University, Fullerton, Los Angeles, California, USA

AUTHORS

MARIE BOLTZ, PhD, CRNP
Professor, Pennsylvania State University, College of Nursing, University Park, Pennsylvania, USA

AMY CAMERON, PA-C
Department of Emergency Medicine, Massachusetts General Hospital, Boston, Massachusetts, USA

CHRISTOPHER R. CARPENTER, MD, MSc, FACEP, AGSF
Professor of Emergency Medicine, Washington University School of Medicine, Emergency Care Research Core, St Louis, Missouri, USA

STEVEN C. CASTLE, MD
Professor of Geriatric Medicine, UCLA School of Medicine, Clinical Director of Geriatrics, VA Greater Los Angeles, CEO and President, DrBalance, Inc, Certified FallProof! Instructor, California State University, Fullerton, Los Angeles, California, USA

RAMON CUEVAS-TRISAN, MD
Chief, Physical Medicine and Rehabilitation Service, West Palm Beach VA Medical Center, University of Miami Miller School of Medicine, Nova Southeastern University College of Osteopathic Medicine, West Palm Beach, Florida, USA

VIKTORIYA FRIDMAN, DNP, RN, ANP-BC
Clinical Professor, Hunter-Bellevue School of Nursing, New York, New York, USA

MICHELLE A. FRITSCH, PharmD
Founder and President, Meds MASH, LLC, Monkton, Maryland, USA

DAVID A. GANZ, MD, PhD
VA Greater Los Angeles Healthcare System, Associate Professor of Medicine, David Geffen School of Medicine at UCLA, Los Angeles, California, USA

ANNA LUCY HATTON, PhD, BSc(Hons)
Senior Lecturer in Physiotherapy, School of Health and Rehabilitation Sciences, University of Queensland, Brisbane, Queensland, Australia

CYNTHIA L. HOLLE, DNP, MBA, RN
Center of Innovation in Long-Term Services and Supports, Providence VA Medical Center, Providence, Rhode Island, USA

JILL KAMINSKI, MS
Clinical Data and Systems Analyst, AvaSure, LLC, Belmont, Michigan, USA

JENNIFER H. LeLAURIN, MPH
Health Science Specialist, Center of Innovation on Disability and Rehabilitation Research (CINDRR), Malcom Randall VA Medical Center, Gainesville, Florida, USA

SHAN LIU, MD, SD, FACEP
Clinical Instructor, Harvard Medical School, Department of Emergency Medicine, Massachusetts General Hospital, Boston, Massachusetts, USA

PATRICIA A. QUIGLEY, PhD, MPH, MS
Nurses Consultant, LLC, St Petersburg, Florida, USA

BARBARA RESNICK, PhD, CRNP
Professor, University of Maryland School of Nursing, Baltimore, Maryland, USA

KEITH ROME, PhD, MSc, BSc (Hons)
Professor of Podiatry, Head of Research, School of Clinical Sciences, Auckland University of Technology, Auckland, New Zealand

JAMES L. RUDOLPH, MD, SM
Center of Innovation in Long-Term Services and Supports, Providence VA Medical Center, Department of Medicine, The Warren Alpert Medical School of Brown University, Center of Gerontology and Health Research, Brown University School of Public Health, Providence, Rhode Island, USA

PENNY S. SHELTON, PharmD
Executive Director, North Carolina Association of Pharmacists, Durham, North Carolina, USA

RONALD I. SHORR, MD, MS, FACP
Director, Geriatric Research Education and Clinical Center (GRECC), Research Professor of Epidemiology, University of Florida, Malcom Randall VA Medical Center, Gainesville, Florida, USA

ANDREA YEVCHAK SILLNER, PhD, GCNS-BC, RN
Center of Innovation in Long-Term Services and Supports, Providence VA Medical Center, Providence, Rhode Island, USA; College of Nursing, The Pennsylvania State University, University Park, Pennsylvania, USA

LISBETH VOTRUBA, MSN, RN
VP of Clinical Quality and Innovation, AvaSure, LLC, Belmont, Michigan, USA

Contents

Public health messaging campaigns stating that falls are bad and can be prevented are not effective, as evidenced by a 30% increase in death from falls over the past decade. A first approach is to use measures of balance to show the magnitude of the problem. Second, the role of ageism as a barrier to required behavioral change should be addressed. Third, explanations should be provided regarding why mobility and balance have changed. As a counter to ageism, pros and cons for specific interventions and how these maximize momentum and mobility should be discussed.

Footwear is a modifiable risk factor for falls in older adults, including populations with metabolic disease, inflammatory arthritis, and neurodegenerative disease. Ill-fitting footwear, and specific design features, such as elevated heels and backless styles, can impair balance control and heighten the risk of falling. Although foot care is routine practice for some older adults to prevent ulceration (eg, diabetes) or relieve symptoms (eg, foot pain), new footwear interventions are emerging with the potential to ameliorate balance and walking impairments. Multifaceted podiatric interventions, which include appropriate footwear and importantly patient education, may have the capacity to reduce falls in older adults.

Falls in the elderly are an increasing problem causing a high degree of morbidity, mortality, and use of health care services. Identification of risk factors through medical assessment supports the provision of appropriate interventions that reduce rates of falling. Evaluation and intervention strategies are generally challenging because of the complex and multifactorial nature of falls. The clinician should consider screening for falls an important part of the functional evaluation in older adults. Several potential interventions have proven helpful as preventive strategies. Optimal approaches involve interdisciplinary collaboration in assessment and interventions, particularly exercise, attention to coexisting medical conditions, and reduction of environmental hazards.

an overview of falls and physical activity prevalence among acute care patients, challenges to engaging patients in physical activity and falls prevention activities and innovative approaches to increase physical activity and prevent falls among older hospitalized patients.

Patient-engaged video surveillance implemented in 71 hospitals over 1 year revealed low rates in assisted and unassisted falls, room elopement, and line, tube, or drain dislodgement per 1000 days of surveillance. Monitor technicians interacted 20.5 times per day with patients who fell and initiated alarms for urgent unit staff response 2.38 times per day, and this accounted for the low fall rate (1.50 falls/1000 days of surveillance) in an adult population. Data on adverse events and timeliness of nursing response to actual urgent and emergent patient conditions provides evidence of the rapid contribution of patient-engaged video surveillance to patient safety.

Through education, frontline nurse involvement, and redesigning fall prevention approach, hourly rounding was promoted as a proactive falls prevention strategy with the goal of decreasing falls and promoting patient safety, health, and comfort. Nurses in health care organizations increase patient safety and reduce patient falls in the hospital setting through hourly rounding with a purpose. Current practices must be redesigned to ensure that acute care fall prevention initiatives are consistent and transformational.

Falls in hospitalized patients are a pressing patient safety concern, but there is a limited body of evidence demonstrating the effectiveness of commonly used fall prevention interventions in hospitals. This article reviews common study designs and the evidence for various hospital fall prevention interventions. There is a need for more rigorous research on fall prevention in the hospital setting.

CLINICS IN GERIATRIC MEDICINE

SERIES OF RELATED INTEREST

Medical Clinics of North America
Primary Care: Clinics in Office Practice
Physical Medicine and Rehabilitation Clinics

THE CLINICS ARE AVAILABLE ONLINE!
Access your subscription at:
www.theclinics.com

Erratum

The article titled "Cognitive Frailty: mechanisms, tools to measure, prevention and controversy" published in August 2017 (Volume 33, Issue 3) has been retracted at the request of the Publisher. This article was plagiarised from the following sources:

1. Ruan Q, Yu Z, Chen M, Bao Z, Li J, He W. Cognitive frailty, a novel target for the prevention of elderly dependency. Ageing research reviews. 2015;20:1-10.
2. Kelaiditi E, Cesari M, Canevelli M, van Kan GA, Ousset PJ, Gillette-Guyonnet S, et al. Cognitive frailty: rational and definition from an (I.A.N.A./I.A.G.G.) international consensus group. The journal of nutrition, health & aging. 2013;17(9):726-34.
3. Halil M, Cemal Kizilarslanoglu M, Emin Kuyumcu M, Yesil Y, Cruz Jentoft AJ. Cognitive aspects of frailty: mechanisms behind the link between frailty and cognitive impairment. The journal of nutrition, health & aging. 2015;19(3):276-83.
4. Robertson DA, Savva GM, Kenny RA. Frailty and cognitive impairment–a review of the evidence and causal mechanisms. Ageing research reviews. 2013;12(4):840-51.
5. Panza F, Solfrizzi V, Barulli MR, Santamato A, Seripa D, Pilotto A, et al. Cognitive Frailty: A Systematic Review of Epidemiological and Neurobiological Evidence of an Age-Related Clinical Condition. Rejuvenation research. 2015;18(5):389-412.
6. Del Campo N, Payoux P, Djilali A, Delrieu J, Hoogendijk EO, Rolland Y, et al. Relationship of regional brain beta-amyloid to gait speed. Neurology. 2016;86(1):36-43.
7. Buchman AS, Schneider JA, Leurgans S, Bennett DA. Physical frailty in older persons is associated with Alzheimer disease pathology. Neurology. 2008;71(7):499-504.
8. Panza F, Solfrizzi V, Giannini M, Seripa D, Pilotto A, Logroscino G. Nutrition, frailty, and Alzheimer's disease. Frontiers in aging neuroscience. 2014;6:221.
9. Robertson DA, Savva GM, Kenny RA. Frailty and cognitive impairment–a review of the evidence and causal mechanisms. Ageing research reviews. 2013;12(4):840-51.
10. Fougere B. Management of Frailty: Screening and Interventions. Journal Nutrition Health and Ageing. [Epub ahead of print].
11. GARN Network's "Whitebook on Frailty."
12. Canevelli M, Cesari M. Cognitive frailty: what is still missing? The journal of nutrition, health & aging. 2015;19(3):273-5.

Of the above sources listed, the following were not included in the authors' reference list:

Ruan Q, Yu Z, Chen M, Bao Z, Li J, He W. Cognitive frailty, a novel target for the prevention of elderly dependency. Ageing research reviews. 2015;20:1-10.

Halil M, Cemal Kizilarslanoglu M, Emin Kuyumcu M, Yesil Y, Cruz Jentoft AJ. Cognitive aspects of frailty: mechanisms behind the link between frailty and cognitive impairment. The journal of nutrition, health & aging. 2015;19(3):276-83.

Panza F, Solfrizzi V, Barulli MR, Santamato A, Seripa D, Pilotto A, et al. Cognitive Frailty: A Systematic Review of Epidemiological and Neurobiological Evidence of an Age-Related Clinical Condition. Rejuvenation research. 2015;18(5):389-412.

Clin Geriatr Med 35 (2019) ix–x
https://doi.org/10.1016/j.cger.2019.01.001
0749-0690/19/© 2019 Published by Elsevier Inc.

Panza F, Solfrizzi V, Giannini M, Seripa D, Pilotto A, Logroscino G. Nutrition, frailty, and Alzheimer's disease. Frontiers in aging neuroscience. 2014;6:221.

Fougere B. Management of Frailty: Screening and Interventions. Journal Nutrition Health and Ageing. [Epub ahead of print]

The GARN Network's "Whitebook on Frailty"

Canevelli M, Cesari M. Cognitive frailty: what is still missing? The journal of nutrition, health & aging. 2015;19(3):273-5.

Preface

New Strategies for Falls Prevention

Despite committed effort of our nation's experts to develop falls prevention strategies to address this major public health issue for older adults, death from falls continues to increase, by 30% over the past decade. Projections suggest that by 2030 seven older adults will die from a fall every hour (https://www.cdc.gov/homeandrecreationalsafety/falls/adultfalls.html). This issue of *Clinics of Geriatric Medicine* is meant to help health care stop doing what is not working and instead pivot to develop better "behaviors" to address this crisis. To do so, I have pulled together an innovative, multidisciplinary team to brainstorm on new approaches and to help identify our common practices that just do not work. It is an honor to be associated with these authors, who I have personally learned from over the years. These ideas, together with new opportunities presented by the Centers for Medicare and Medicaid Services of implementing supplemental benefits to support wellness approaches to health, should facilitate providers and health plans to implement changes to help older adults maximize their mobility, social engagement, and independence.

This review on falls prevention does not address approaches in the outpatient setting, but the ongoing Patient-Centered Outcomes Research Institute (PCORI)/National Institute on Aging Strategies To Reduce Injuries and Develop Confidence in Elders (STRIDE) should provide much needed input in the near future on changing our approach to falls risk in primary care, and resources to start are on the STRIDE Web site (http://www.stride-study.org/). In discussing needed behavior change in outpatient settings, my article, entitled "Despite Active Public Health Campaigns, Death from Falls Increased 30% in the Past Decade: Is Ageism Part of the Barrier to Self-Awareness?," addresses the potential role of ageism in the inadequate response to current national campaigns to address falls as well and suggests an approach to counseling that can be included in the medical decision-making component of progress notes to warrant higher level of evaluation and management (E/M) codes. My article tries to provide a theoretical framework as to how ageism could be a significant driver in the challenge of getting those most at risk of injury to make the needed behavior changes to avoid injury from falls. However, there is a unifying theme that has to do with the role of motivational interviewing techniques to support needed health-behavior changes. Drs Resnick and Boltz (in their article, "Optimizing Function and Physical Activity in Hospitalized Older Adults to Prevent Functional Decline and Falls," discussed more later) address this well in their review on the need to improve physical activity in the inpatient setting.

The article, by Hatton and Rome, on age-related changes in feet and footwear emphasizes an important, often overlooked perspective of falls risk and an excellent

Clin Geriatr Med 35 (2019) xi–xiv
https://doi.org/10.1016/j.cger.2019.02.001
0749-0690/19/© 2019 Published by Elsevier Inc.

starting point for behavior change. This article reviews gender differences and age-related disease changes in feet with critical information to individualize management based on underlying chronic conditions, and a final call to develop more innovative footwear to address both comfort and balance in older adults to literally maximize their mobility. Later, when we address hospital falls, a common and entrenched "check-the-box" approach to falls risk management is to use nonskid socks, which actually is the single greatest risk of falls,[1] and this is addressed in Drs Hatton and Rome's article. The article by Dr Cuevas-Trisan is a review on balance problems and falls, which can also help the primary care provider address medical complexity and potential diagnoses to enhance E/M billing codes to improve reimbursement. The article by Fritsch and Shelton suggests a novel approach for pharmacists to function as "brokers," in addition to the more traditional role of medication reconciler and reviewer of potential adverse effects of falls risk–inducing medications, or FRIDs. The role of medications in falls is not new, but the current older adult population is likely to be on more medications than similarly aged older adults a decade ago due to guidelines in chronic disease management and advances in pharmaceuticals in general. Hence, the broker role, of being more direct in assessment and then making referrals back to primary care providers or consultants, and with a newer dynamic suggested of referring to physical therapy/occupational therapy or home improvement contractors. The article provides a practical six-step approach that starts with basic structured observational gait, and the pharmacist's role as broker is boosted by doing simple screening assessments recommended in primary care by the Centers for Disease Control and Prevention.

The article by Dr Carpenter and colleagues addresses the opportunities and challenges of addressing falls in the context of the Emergency Department (ED). It touches on "preacute" falls risk assessments and the challenges and lack of evidence of doing this using Emergency Management Services. One option not discussed is to implement this through other "eyes-on" home services, such as Meals on Wheels, direct care workers, or transportation services. The article discusses the challenges of risk assessment that they take time to do once the patient is in the ED, as most tools were developed for other settings, and the interest, focus, and training of ED staff often do not include falls risk assessment, changes in mobility with aging, or knowledge of community-based resources. The other complexity touched on in the ED setting and discussed in depth in the article by Sillner and colleagues is the interaction between falls and delirium. The other option is the referral after the ED visit to a community falls clinic; the article states that there are 23 such entities in the Netherlands. Wonder how many there are in the United States? However, it discusses how there is low compliance with follow-up and identifies transportation issues and disinterest in following up, which is likely due to unrecognized self-ageism (discussed in my article in this issue) or cognitive decline. Finally, this article provides a nice overview of the potential of technology to support preacute recognition of changes in mobility or balance, including the Apple 4 watch. The challenge of this approach is discussed, including the high false-negative and false-positive response and the challenge of interface with health care (who gets the alerts and how do you respond?).

The next series of articles addresses falls risk in the inpatient setting with excellent literature reviews on preventing falls and addressing the complex interaction of delirium and falls in the inpatient setting. A common theme discussed is how much of the published literature is primarily on quality improvement projects that share the challenge in rigorously defining the intervention and the methods of implementation, making dissemination very difficult. Of note, evidence-based approaches to reduce injuries from falls are still lacking, as this is still considered an "emerging science" despite the longstanding significance. The hallmark of delirium impacts crucial inpatient environmental factors, including tethers (catheters, IVs, monitors), awareness of strength and balance decline, low lighting, and awareness of "where is the bathroom," which is similar to getting up in the middle of the night in a motel but further complicated by illness. These articles provide support for improving quality improvement efforts. Methods for detection/defining and inclusion of delirium are therefore tantamount in quality improvement projects moving forward. The following quality improvement review articles provide a strong basis for inclusion in adopting a different behavior with detailed discussion of components and implementation on true "culture changes" needed in taking a different approach to falls in the inpatient setting:

1. Optimizing function and physical activity (Resnick and Boltz)
2. A review of large-scale use of patient-engaged video surveillance (Quigley and colleagues)
3. Key concepts for implementing intentional rounding with a focus on toileting (Fridman)

The article in this issue by LeLaurin and Schorr, "Preventing Falls in Hospitalized Patients: State of the Science," is a critical review of the evidence in preventing falls in the hospital summary and is the anchor to this issue. After reviewing these quality improvement promising practices, it is important to reflect on the evidence-based reviews of Sillner and colleagues and LeLaurin and Schorr. Of note, the review on delirium and falls identified a relative risk of delirium associated with falls being 4.5 (1.4-12.6) and that these two outcomes are inextricably linked. Therefore, improved screening and detection of delirium should be included in any quality improvement project to address the relevance of inclusion of delirium in any falls prevention intervention moving forward. This requires active team engagement between nursing, therapy, pharmacy, and hospitalists.

What is missing from this "call to a different approach" to help older adults maximize mobility are reviews of exercise interventions. A recent network meta-analysis identified exercise interventions as the most important to reduce injury from falls and that the combination of an exercise intervention plus screening and addressing vision changes resulted in 97% reduced risk of injury from falls.[2] The challenge is to understand and build the right type, intensity, and frequency (dose) of exercise that is crucial but is currently not defined; awareness of what is available and what is the quality of community-based programs is beyond the scope of most providers/health plans. As the PCORI/STRIDE project continues, it is hoped we will gain more information and help with how to approach this issue. Again, with broadening of Medicare Advantage supplement benefits to support wellness programs being rolled out in 2019 and 2020, there is significant opportunity for health plans to bridge this crucial gap with community-based exercise programs and provide the needed support to tailor ongoing exercise to older adults with varying chronic conditions. Likewise, the "It Takes a Village" approach means better interaction between exercise programs, primary care, physical therapy, subspecialists (back, shoulder, knee), and perhaps a new role for pharmacists as "broker." Let's get at it!

Steven C. Castle, MD
Geriatric Medicine
UCLA School of Medicine
VA Greater Los Angeles
DrBalance, Inc
California State University
Fullerton, 11301 Wilshire Blvd
GRECC 11G Bld 158 Rm 117
Los Angeles, CA 90073, USA

E-mail address:
scastle@gravity-happens.com

REFERENCES

1. Koepsell TD, Wolf ME, Buchner DM, et al. Footwear style and risk of falls in older adults. J Am Geriatr Soc 2004;52:1495–501.
2. Tricco AC, Thomas SM, Veroniki AA, et al. Comparisons of interventions for preventing falls in older adults a systematic review and meta-analysis. JAMA 2017; 318:1687–99.

Despite Active Public Health Campaigns, Death from Falls Increased 30% in the Past Decade

Is Ageism Part of the Barrier to Self-Awareness?

Steven C. Castle, MD

KEYWORDS

- Mobility and balance • Postural control • Injury from falls • Ageism
- Multisensory integration

KEY POINTS

- Current public health messaging campaigns stating (1) falls are bad and (2) falls can be prevented has not worked, as evidenced by a 30% increase in death from falls over the past decade.
- Ageism has been shown to contribute to a significant impact on health including shorter life expectancy, early cardiovascular events, less adoption of healthy behaviors, poor recovery from illness or injury, and increased risk of dementia.
- Ageism is a likely contributor to the barrier of recognizing common mobility and balance changes as we age, and is part of the reason of the failure of current public health messaging on falls.
- Ageism can have a broad impact on altering postural control response to loss of balance, and may manifest as delayed or ineffective multisensory integration of postural control.
- Ageism is a likely contributor to low uptake of specific behaviors proved to reduce injury from falls including exercise, use of mobility aids, home modification, and seeking assistance.

Because falls are the largest public health issues for older adults, significant efforts at addressing this problem have been led by the Centers for Disease Control and Prevention (CDC) STEADI (Stopping Elderly Accidents, Deaths, and Injuries) program and The National Council On Aging (NCOA) evidence-based list of programs.[1,2] The NCOA supports "the expansion and sustainability of evidence-based health promotion and

Disclosure: S.C. Castle provides consultation, training, and solutions to address common changes in mobility and balance of older adults in health care practices, acute care, long-term care, older adult communities, and in the home.
UCLA School of Medicine, VA Greater Los Angeles, DrBalance, Inc, California State University, Fullerton, 11301 Wilshire Blvd, GRECC 11G Bld 158 Rm 117, Los Angeles, CA 90073, USA
E-mail address: scastle@gravity-happens.com

disease prevention programs in the community and online through collaboration with national, state, and community partners." In 2005, the NCOA led the development of the Falls Free National Action Plan and updated this strategy in 2015, with specific goals and strategies to effect sustained initiatives that reduce falls among older adults. The objective was to "reduce the rate of emergency department visits due to falls among older adults by 10%." The CDC STEADI initiative "offers a coordinated approach to implementing the American and British Geriatrics Societies' Clinical Practice Guideline for fall prevention."[3] The STEADI program consists of 3 core elements of screening falls risk, assessment of modifiable risk factors, and interventions to reduce identified risk factors. Many national experts in falls prevention participated in both these efforts.

Despite these efforts, recent data from the *Morbidity and Mortality Weekly Report* says that death from falls has increased 30% over the past decade,[4] despite a recent network meta-analysis stating that injury from falls can be reduced by 98% if older adults engage in a mobility and balance exercise intervention together with screening and treatment of underlying vision problems.[5] Perhaps we should better understand the limitations of the current approach and consider alternative strategies. This position paper will provide evidence for one of the barriers that needs to be addressed to be effective, namely, the role of ageism in creating barriers to self-awareness and the adoption of needed preventive behavior strategies that have demonstrated efficacy at reducing injury and deaths from falls. This article reviews theoretic models of how ageism could be contributing to the apparent lack of efficacy of current public health strategies for the prevention of falls.

Studies from a decade ago identified barriers to success of traditional efforts of falls prevention campaigns. The traditional strategy is to highlight 2 concepts: (1) falls are a significant health issue and (2) there is strong evidence that falls and, in particular, injury from falls can be prevented, which is seen in the most recent CDC post.[6] Studies looking at the uptake of this message have shown that older adults perceive this to be an issue for frail older adults (which they have great difficulty in identifying with this cohort) and that falls are accidental and not preventable.[7] The key barrier is the lack of personal relevance to the group that is most affected by this public health issue.

SIGNIFICANT IMPACT ON HEALTH AND WELLNESS FROM AGEISM

Ageism, the bias against older adults and the natural aging process, has been identified and remains the most condoned and prevalent form of discrimination,[8] and is prevalent in our media.[9] Much research has demonstrated the significant negative impact of ageism over the life course. Younger older adults who express a positive self-perception of aging have on average a 7.6-year increased longevity compared with older adults with a negative self-perception of aging.[10] The mechanism to this is related to lifestyle choices and healthy behaviors. Of 8 identified preventive healthy behaviors ranked 1 to 5 (from "not adopted" to "very important to adopt"), those that had a positive self-perception of aging scored significantly higher on the importance of these behaviors.[11] This effect is over the life course, and negative stereotype beliefs predict early mortality from cardiovascular disease 30 years after the attitudes were measured.[12] Positive beliefs toward aging are also associated with higher hippocampal volumes ($P<.007$) and fewer plaques and tangles ($P = .026$) and a lower incidence of dementia diagnosis in all participants and even in those at increased risk for apolipoprotein E ε4.[13,14]

So how can ageism affect the hidden public health problem of continued increase in injury and deaths from falls despite strong evidence that injury from falls can be prevented, and the existence of significant policy efforts to reduce them? First, the physiologic components that are involved in balance control response are reviewed (**Fig. 1**), followed by a discussion of how ageism might be affecting these responses (**Figs. 2 and 3**).

BRIEF REVIEW OF BALANCE CONTROL PHYSIOLOGY

Postural control involves sensory input, sensory integration, and motor response[15] (see **Fig. 1**). Sensory postural control involves distinct input routes, including vision, somatosensory, and vestibular. As a person encounters an obstacle or loss of balance as determined by the sensory inputs, this information is integrated (multisensory integration [MSI]) involving cortical (frontal/prefrontal and parietal), cerebellar, and vestibular input, which is transmitted and further processed in the basal ganglia.[16] Signals for a motor response are then transmitted down the spinal column, and the balance control motor responses have been described as an ankle, hip, or step/grasp response. The response results in balance recovery or a fall. If a fall occurs, an individual might be motivated to understand what caused the loss of balance, and what approaches could mitigate future fall events. This latter concept is really at the heart of the CDC STEADI approach to properly assess for individual risk factors and then develop interventions to address the identified risk factors.

Fig. 1B shows how 75% of older adults have slower univariate sensory reaction time that requires MSI support, but these individuals had worse balance (uniped stance) with higher rates of falls, perhaps because of decline in motor response performance and lack of adaptation of appropriate behaviors.[17] This suggests a psychophysical integrative difference in postural control of older adults, and the potential impact of ageism has not been studied.

Ageism could be a key influence on the poor self-awareness of falls risk or balance control response in older adults. How poor response to falls prevention efforts fits the

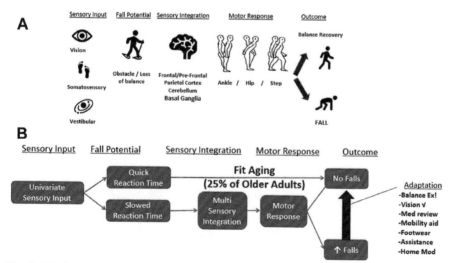

Fig. 1. (*A*) Overview of postural control physiology. (*B*) Psychophysical integrative differences with aging in postural control response.

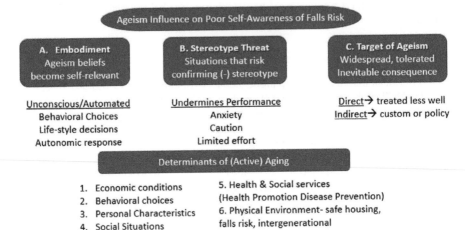

Fig. 2. Risk of ageism model. (*Data from* Nelson TD. Ageism: prejudice against our feared future self. J Soc Issues 2005;61(2):207–21.)

Risk of Ageism Model (RAM) is briefly reviewed[18] here and is presented in **Fig. 2**. The RAM states that 3 processes, (A) Ageism Embodiment, (B) Ageism Threat, and (C) Target of Ageism, result in a negative influence of determinants of active aging. The specific impact on falls prevention efforts are described later.

POTENTIAL INFLUENCE OF AGING ON POOR SELF-AWARENESS OF FALLS

Again, ageism could be manifested as poor self-awareness of falls risk through 3 methods of influence: embodiment, stereotype threat, and actual targets of ageism (direct and indirect). Embodied cognition relates to how the mind and body are inter-twined.[19] The effects of ageism could be manifested through physical changes involving neuromuscular speed (reaction time) and gait and balance performance. It could also manifest through cognitive changes resulting in slowdowns, especially in visuospatial processing and MSI. Finally, how societal factors are influencing these

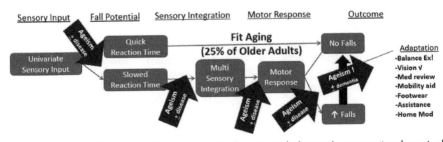

Fig. 3. Adverse effect of ageism + chronic disease and dementia on postural control response.

responses have largely gone unstudied but are likely to be significant, based on the impact of ageism on other health/disease states that have been studied.

Embodied Cognition

Embodied cognition is a broad theoretic framework for understanding the intertwining of mind-body relations, and specifically that higher-level cognition (ie, impact of ageism) is grounded in sensorimotor processing that is so crucial to postural control and mobility.[19] Ageism is the most condoned and accepted form of discrimination in our society, is prevalent throughout our media and written language, and affects everyone across the age course.[8,20] The inevitability of aging means that most people's negative attitude toward aging eventually becomes self-relevant. Prior papers have discussed the impact on health and in particular the impact on factors associated with active aging. What has been underappreciated is how this may be affecting the continued escalation in injuries from falls, and in particular deaths from falls. The impact of ageism on embodied cognition may result in an impaired physiologic response in postural control.

Sensory perception and integration

Significant work has been done on sensory perception and integration as it relates to balance. Potential ageism impact may relate to the identified visual dominance of older adults, who rely less on somatosensory input. Older adults have been found to look at the ground more than younger adults.[21] A key study identified that 25% of older adults (mean age 75.1 ± 6.3 years, 57% female) demonstrate univariate (vision or somatosensory) rapid reaction time equivalent to that of younger adults, or what could be called "fit" older adults.[17] These individuals did not need or benefit from MSI of other sensory inputs (combined vision and somatosensory). The other 75% did demonstrate improved reaction time through MSI, although this group had a significantly higher fall rate (42% versus 17%, $P\leq.05$) and diminished uniped stance time (13.2 ± 10.8 versus 21.4 ± 11.6 seconds, $P<.01$). The research questions include "can those who have slowed univariate and reliance on MSI but are more prone to falls be identified," and/or "can improvement in MSI reaction time be demonstrated by balance training," such as through the FallProof! method that specifically focuses on training in MSI processes.[15]

Body schema and peripersonal space

The capacity to perform an action requires an awareness of one's body within the surrounding external space, which is continually updated by vestibular signals.[22] Given the common changes in vestibular function with aging, it is anticipated a significant age effect could be demonstrated, especially among inactive older adults. This could be reflected in age-related changes in mental imagery. Older adults have a decline especially in mental perceptions of body rotation.[19] An example of this was in a study of older adults (mean age 75.4 ± 5.5 years) on walking an instrumented course and demonstrated greater error in estimating turn exit points (versus observers and instrumentation): the greater the discrepancy, the more impaired was visuospatial performance.[23] Another example of age-related changes in body schema was a study that documented motor cautiousness in older adults' shoulder rotation movements when walking through door frames.[24] It is hypothesized that negative attitudes about aging be correlated with this increased cautiousness even in a commonly encountered movement.

Ageism Threat

Stereotype threat refers to a threat experienced by an individual when they are in a situation that puts them at risk of confirming a negative stereotype about themselves.

Because ageism is embodied, being presented with a situation that consciously or subconsciously exposes such bias results in a response of anxiety, caution, or limited effort that undermines performance.[18] This may explain why those with balance changes with aging do not choose to participate in the most effective intervention in preventing injury from falls, namely balance exercises.[25] Specifically, ageism-stigmatized individuals avoid a negative experience of stereotype threat by not engaging in the most recommended preventive experience to reduce injury from falls.[18] An example of how this ageism threat affects performance is now discussed.

Perceived threat impact on performance that relates to postural control

A study demonstrated how perceived stress could blunt dual-task balance tasks via measurable blunting of brain activity in the prefrontal cortex (PFC) response to the dual task of walking while talking (WWT). This blunting of the PFC response to a dual task is a perfect example of how embodied cognition may play a key role in cognitive control, especially under attention-demanding conditions, with the measurable decline in gait performance under dual tasks such as WWT, known as the dual-task cost.[26] Those with high dual tasks costs on balance control have demonstrated the increased risk of both cognitive decline and falls risk years down the road in those that exhibit high dual-task costs.[27] This study looked at those without evidence of cognitive decline but rated the stress associated with the dual task (rated as 0 to 10, 10 being very stressful) while walking on an instrumented course while stating every other letter starting with the letter "B." Participants were a mean age 76.8 ± 6.7 years and were 56% female. While walking the course, oxygenation of the PFC was measured using functional near-infrared spectroscopy, which was quantified as oxygenated hemoglobin (Hbo_2). Results revealed that higher perceived stress was associated with greater decline in stride velocity (dual-task cost) in moving from single to dual-task conditions, which was associated with a blunted increase in Hbo_2 in the PFC, but in men only.[26]

Perceived threat impact on perception and action

Perceptual scaling of tasks has found that older adult are sensitive to environmental impediments that complicate walking, such as crossing a river by walking across stepping stones (personal experience of the author). Older adults when standing at the bottom of a hill and asked to estimate the slope of various angled hills perceive the slope as steeper than younger counterparts.[28] Other estimates of other environmental impediments indicate increased cautiousness of older adults, consistent with the stereotype threat theory.[19] What would be interesting is to measure perceived attitudes toward aging to discover whether there is a correlation between perceived slope estimates and cautiousness.

Target of Ageism

Age discrimination is prevalent in settings where older people can be excluded or denied access to a product, service, or treatment, such as employment or in health and social care. Direct discrimination occurs because of age, whereas indirect discrimination occurs because of custom, policy, or established practice. An analogy to indirect discrimination is a set of steps to enter a building, which denies access to those with reduced functional capacity to climb stairs.[18] Age discrimination is prevalent in the Entertainment and Media industry. A study of the presence and portrayal of older adults in the 50 most popular television series (for viewers aged both 18–49 and 65 and older) between June 1, 2016 and May 31, 2017 was conducted by the University of Southern California Annenberg Inclusion Initiative. Of the 72 unique shows identified, only 9.4% of the speaking parts were age 60 and older. Of the 121 writers of these 72 episodes, 5% were age 60 or older, and of the 100 showrunners, 11% were age 60 and older. Shows without a writer age 60+ had ageism content 81.2% of the time versus ageist content of only 18.8% with a writer age 60+. The same held true for showrunners, with 75% ageist content if no showrunner age 60+ versus 25% with older showrunners.[29] The technology industry also threatens to ramp up ageism, as seen with the quote that "while lycra and yoga make 50 the new 30, technology threatens to make 30 the new 50," especially with media being targeted to handheld devices for this market.[30]

A longitudinal study from the nationally represented Health and Retirement Study (administered in 2008 with follow-up through 2012) specifically identified discrimination in health care delivery, defined as perception of receiving "poorer service or treatment than other people from doctors or hospitals," and the frequency rated as never, infrequent (less than once a year), or frequent (more than once a year).[31] The mean age was 67 years, 83.1% were white, and 56.3% were female. Experience of health care discrimination was reported at 18.6%, with 12.6% being infrequent and 5.9% being frequent. The most common reasons for discrimination were age (28%), gender (12%), and financial status (12%). Almost one-third of participants (29%) who experienced health care discrimination developed new or worsening disability over the next 4 years, compared with 16.8% of those with infrequent or 14.7% of those who never experienced health care discrimination ($P<.001$), with an adjusted hazard ratio of new or worsened disability over 4 years of 1.63 (95% CI, 1.16 to 2.27).

Impact of Ageism on Mobility and Balance/Falls Risk

To sum up, **Fig. 1**A shows the physiologic postural control response and **Fig. 1**B shows the shift in the measured response in 75% of healthy older adults, with slower reaction time requiring more input from MSI but a higher rate of falls than seen in the rapid univariate reaction time of "fit" older adults.[17] **Fig. 2** shows the RAM with the 3 methods of influence of ageism, (A) Embodiment, (B) Ageism Threat, and (C) Target of Ageism.[18] **Fig. 3** ties these 2 concepts together, showing how ageism and/or chronic disease could jeopardize the physiologic postural control response. The initial shift toward slowed reaction time could be due to all 3 methods of ageism, with behavioral choices to not engage in exercise or balance risk exposure, resulting in poor performance resulting from caution or anxiety (as demonstrated in the study that showed less oxygenation in the PFC in older adults who perceived the dual walking task as more stressful[26]). An example of being the target of ageism is commonly seen in older adult communities, where falls are often hid and not addressed because of prevalent ageism as well as fear of losing independent living status.[32] Abnormal autonomic response as a result of embodiment of aging could result in increased heart rate and activation of the hypothalamic-pituitary-adrenal axis that may result in a slowed MSI processing as a result of changes in the PFC influence on the basal ganglia.[26]

Reframing Aging—the FrameWorks Institute Approach: Application to Falls

The FrameWorks Institute, funded by The John A. Hartford Foundation and in association with 7 aging-focused national organizations, carried out empirical testing of approaches to improve messaging on aging that countered the implicit bias of "fighting" or "battling" aging. In testing shifts in implicit attitudes, through focus groups and surveys involving more than 10,000 participants, the metaphor of "building momentum" changes how people understand aging and helps them see how the force of experience and wisdom enables older people to improve their communities[33] (http://www.frameworksinstitute.org/aging.html). Although this Reframing Aging project did not specifically address falls or response to falls risk, perhaps adopting this strategy might be more effective than the approach that (1) falls are bad and (2) falls can be prevented; currently the basis of the major public health approaches of the CDC and NCOA.

Ernest Hemingway in *The Sun Also Rises* states there are 2 ways a person can become bankrupt, gradually and all at once. This is analogous to how falls often present. To better address this, we can use the "maximize momentum" metaphor to supplant the need for self-awareness of falls risk (falls are bad) and preventive steps to avoid the consequences of falls (falls can be prevented). This supports the concept of maintaining independence and mobility by making choices that help sustain and maximize momentum for as long as possible.

Maximize Momentum as We Age!

Seek to identify changes in your mobility,

Ask why, and develop strategies to

Maximize momentum for independence and mobility

Be able to go where you want to go!

TAKING A DIFFERENT APPROACH

Older adults downplay both the personal risk of falls and when a fall does occur. There is much embarrassment when a fall occurs, and often humor is used in an attempt to cover such embarrassment. There is also a concern of losing independence if falls are reported, with family and doctors recommending a higher level of care. This is certainly true in older adult communities with concern of moving from independent to assisted or skilled levels of care, and where ageism is often felt most strongly, ironically enough.[32] Older adults frequently do not discuss falls with their doctor unless an injury occurs, partly because doctors do not pay much attention to falls unless an injury does occur. Both often take the approach that you need to "be more careful" without really getting at potential changes in mobility that are contributing to this and future fall events. Ageism is most likely an undercurrent to this approach from both an older adult and a health care perspective. Falls should not be seen as a harbinger of old age (an ageism perspective) but instead a physiologic change that deserves to be addressed with necessary adaptations. It would be like no longer being able to read because you do not want to look old by having to wear glasses.

One approach is to use a cognitive-based approach to train older adults to improve at dual tasks using computerized cognitive training to improve mobility. A review demonstrated a significant improvement in dual-task walking but not simple gait.[34] However, a more direct approach should be tested using primary care providers to address recognition of and reasons for mobility changes, similarly as has been done with other public health issues such as breast cancer or osteoporosis: specifically, using a team approach with tracking of completion of steps as outlined here.

Measurement of Changes in Balance

Several simple approaches of measuring balance changes that are common can be performed in a variety of settings, and by older adults themselves, as listed in

Table 1. The Senior Fitness Test has the advantage of having percentile rankings by 5-year increments beyond age 60 and gender, to objectively identify reduced fitness compared with age-matched peers.[35] More sophisticated measures such as the Fullerton Advanced Balance Scale (FAB) provide more of an awareness of which components of postural control are not performing as expected.[36]

Measurement of Self-Awareness of Falls Risk

Once it can be determined whether someone's balance and mobility is below average, an approach to self-awareness can be measured.[37,38] Reasons for lack of self-awareness are not clear, nor the approach on how to improve it. Showing results from testing balance and fitness may help, especially as a percentile ranking from the Senior Fitness Test. Lord Kelvin is famous for his quote, "You cannot improve what cannot be measured."

Explore Negative Attitudes Toward Aging as a Variable

Measures of self-perceptions of attitudes toward aging exist and have been correlated with health outcomes, as discussed previously.[39] A small study of 47 older adults (63–82 years) were given a 30-minute video game with either a positive or negative image of aging. Walking speed before/after playing a 30-minute computer game with a positive image of aging showed a 9% significant increase in gait speed, whereas there was no change in speed among those viewing a computer game with a negative stereotype of aging.[40] Perhaps a more direct approach to confronting the decline in initiation of an intervention with proven efficacy in reducing falls would be to address whether the patient has an ageist bias, such as thinking that canes or walkers are for old people. Reframing this from the perspective of a way of maximizing momentum and achieving other desired goals of social engagement may help. A trial of using the analogy of needing to wear glasses to read, and feeling older when wearing them, might help provide some insight.

If a person has low self-awareness of falls risk and declines recommended interventions but is found to have a positive attitude about aging, other confounders should be pursued. If this could be related to cognitive decline, further assessment in that domain is warranted. If it is related to fear of participating in a balance class, more 1-to-1 physical therapy may be warranted. This is particularly true of older adults with very low FAB scores but who have positive attitudes about aging. One approach may be to directly discuss concerns about a possible intervention to improve mobility.

Table 1
Office-based measures of changes in balance and mobility

Maneuver	References
1. Have you had a fall, become fearful of falling, or changed activities because of your balance?	CDC[41]
2. Structured observational gait	Verghese et al,[42] 2009
3. 4-Stage Balance Test	CDC[43]
4. 8-Foot up and go (>8.5 s at risk for falls)	Rose et al,[44] 2002
5. Timed up and go (≥12 s at risk for falls)	CDC[45]
6. 30 s Chair stands (>15 s for 5 is risk for falls)	Zhang et al,[46] 2013; CDC[47]
7. Gait velocity (>1 m/s is normal, <0.7 is abnormal, <0.4 is frail) (decline in 0.1 increased risk of ED admission)	Purser et al,[48] 2005
8. Fullerton Advanced Balance Scale	Hernandez & Rose[36] 2008

Write down possible interventions on a piece of paper or flip chart and list positive and negative reasons for engaging in that option to try and decipher the rationale for reluctance. It is possible that this could be done in a group class or shared medical appointment format.

Provide Explanation of How and Why Balance Has Changed

Provide written information to patients about possible changes in balance control and how possible risky medications might be responsible for changes in mobility. Include discussions about possible risky medications but also the need to control chronic conditions, especially hypertension. If a risky medication is more for control of a symptom rather than a disease (ie, neuropathy), ask how well controlled the neuropathy is; is it 10%, 50%, or 80% better to help engage the patient in decisions to continue or stop a risky medication? Include discussion about any coexisting cognitive decline and how that might be affecting decision making with the patient, spouse, and family.

Use Motivational Interviewing Approach with Specific, Measurable, Achievable, Realistic, and Time frame Goals

Write down on paper the possible interventions to address probable causes for changes in mobility. Discuss barriers to implementing any of the options, and discuss how ageism may be contributing to perceptions, and flip it to discuss the role in maximizing momentum. Provide a ranking of what the doctor recommends and a ranking of what the patient would like to do. If a patient has difficulty relating the discussion to himself or herself, try moving the discussion to concern a third person the patient cares about. Come up with an SMART goal (Specific, Measurable, Achievable, Realistic, and Time frame).

SUMMARY

We should try a different approach because the decade-long effort at using the message that (1) falls are bad and (2) falls can be prevented has not been effective with our current cohort of older adults.[3] One approach is to use measures of balance to show the magnitude of the problem as we do with blood pressure, cholesterol, or blood sugars. A second way is to look for the role of ageism as a bias and barrier and address it head on. A third method is to provide explanations as to why mobility and balance has changed and discuss the pros and cons for specific interventions to adapt and counter these changes to support maximizing momentum and the ability to get to where you want to go. New approaches need to be tested, including group classes and care management using a checklist approach. We can do better.

REFERENCES

1. CDC STEADI program. Available at: https://www.cdc.gov/steadi/. Accessed November 1, 2018.
2. NCOA evidence-based programs. Available at: https://www.ncoa.org/resources/2015-falls-free-national-falls-prevention-action-plan/. Accessed November 1, 2018.
3. Available at: https://www.ncbi.nlm.nih.gov/pubmed/?term=Summary+of+the+Updated+American+Geriatrics+Society%2FBritish. Accessed November 1, 2018.
4. Burns E, Kakara R. Deaths from falls among persons aged ≥65 years—United States, 2007-2016. MMWR Morb Mortal Wkly Rep 2018;67:509–14.
5. Tricco AC, Thomas SM, Veroniki AA, et al. Comparisons of interventions for preventing falls in older adults a systematic review and meta-analysis. JAMA 2017; 318:1687–99.

6. Current CDC message—falls are bad and they can be prevented. Available at: https://www.cdc.gov/homeandrecreationalsafety/falls/index.html. Accessed September 1, 2018.
7. Hughes K, van Beurden E, Eakin EG, et al. Older persons' perception of risk of falling: implications for fall-prevention campaigns. Am J Public Health 2008;98:351–7.
8. Nelson TD. Ageism: prejudice against our feared future self. J Soc Issues 2005; 61(2):207–21.
9. Smith SL, Pieper K, Choueiti M. Still rare, still ridiculed: portrayals of senior characters on screen in popular films from 2015 and 2016. USC Annenberg inclusion initiative. Available at: https://annenberg.usc.edu/sites/default/files/2018/01/22/Still %20Rare%20Still%20Ridiculed%20Final%20Report%20January%202018.pdf. Accessed April 12, 2018.
10. Levy BR, Slade MD, Kunkel SR. Longevity increased by positive self-perceptions of aging. J Pers Soc Psychol 2002;83(2):261–70.
11. Levy BR, Myers LM. Preventive health behaviors influenced by self-perceptions of aging. Prev Med 2004;39:625–9.
12. Levy BR, Zonderman AB, Slade MD, et al. Age stereotypes held earlier in life predict cardiovascular events in later life. Psychol Sci 2009;20(3):296–8.
13. Levy BR, Slade MD, Ferrucci L, et al. A culture-brain link: negative age stereotypes predict Alzheimer's disease biomarkers. Psychol Aging 2016;31(1):82–8.
14. Levy BR, Slade MD, Pietrzak RH, et al. Positive age beliefs protect against dementia even among elders with high-risk gene. PLoS One 2018;13(2):e0191004.
15. Rose DJ. FallProof!™: a comprehensive balance and mobility training program. 2nd edition. Champaign (IL): Human Kinetics; 2010.
16. Holtzer R, Epstein N, Mahoney JR, et al. Neuroimaging of mobility in aging: a targeted review. J Gerontol A Biol Sci Med Sci 2014;69(11):1375–88.
17. Mahoney JR, Holtzer R, Verghese J. Visual-somatosensory integration and balance: evidence for psychophysical integrative differences in aging. Multisens Res 2014;27(1):17–42.
18. Swift HJ, Abrams D. The risks of ageism model: how ageism and negative attitudes toward age can be a barrier to active aging. Soc Issues Policy Rev 2016;1–37.
19. Costello MC, Bloesch EK. Are older adults less embodied? A review of age effects through the lens of embodied cognition. Front Psychol 2017;8:267.
20. Ng R, Allore HG, Trentalange M, et al. Increasing negativity of age stereotypes across 200 years: evidence from a database of 400 million words. PLoS One 2015;10(2):e0117086.
21. Anderson PG, Nienhuis B, Mulder T, et al. Are older adults more dependent on visual information in regulating self-motion than younger adults? J Mot Behav 1998;30:104–13.
22. Lopez C, Schreyer HM, Preuss N, et al. Vestibular stimulation modifies the body schema. Neuropsychologia 2012;50:1830–7.
23. England SE, Verghese J, Mahoney JR, et al. Three-level rating of turns while walking. Gait Posture 2015;41:300–3.
24. Hackney AL, Cinelli MD. Action strategies of older adults walking through apertures. Gait Posture 2011;33:733–6.
25. US Preventive Services Task Force. Falls prevention in older adults: counseling and preventive medication. 2018. Available at: https://www. uspreventiveservicestaskforce.org/Page/Document/UpdateSummaryFinal/falls-prevention-in-older-adults-counseling-and-preventive-medication. Accessed June 1, 2018.

26. Holtzer R, Schoen C, Demetiou E, et al. Stress and gender effects on prefrontal cortex oxygenation levels assessed during single and dual-task walking conditions. Eur J Neurosci 2017;45:660–70.

27. Montero-Odasso M, Verghese J, Beauchet O, et al. Gait and cognition: a complementary approach to understanding brain function and the risk of falling. J Am Geriatr Soc 2012;60:2127–36.

28. Bhalla M, Proffitt DR. Visual-motor recalibration in geographical slant perception. J Exp Psychol Hum Percept Perform 1999;25:1076–96.

29. Smith SL, Pieper K, Choueti. Seniors on the small screen: aging in popular television content. 2017. Available at: http://assets.uscannenberg.org/docs/Seniors_on_the_Small_Screen-Dr_Stacy_L_Smith_9-12-17.pdf. Accessed March 15, 2018.

30. Friend T. Why ageism never gets old. The New Yorker November 20, 2017 issue. 2017. Available at: https://www.newyorker.com/magazine/2017/11/20/why-ageism-never-gets-old. Accessed November 21, 2017.

31. Rogers SE, Thrasher AD, Miao Y, et al. Discrimination in healthcare settings is associated with disability in older adults: health and retirement study, 2008-2012. J Gen Intern Med 2015;30(10):1413–20.

32. Burling S. Old and ageist: why so many older people have prejudices about their peers—and themselves. The Inquirer April 4, 2018. 2018. Available at: http://www.philly.com/philly/health/old-and-ageist-why-do-so-many-older-people-have-prejudices-about-their-peers-and-themselves-20180404.html. Accessed April 7, 2018.

33. FrameWorks institute reframing aging. Available at: http://www.frameworksinstitute.org/aging.html. Accessed May 1, 2015.

34. Marusic U, Vergheses J, Mahoney JR. Cognitive-based interventions to improve mobility: a systematic review and meta-analysis. J Am Med Dir Assoc 2018;19:484–91.

35. Rikli RE, Jone JC. Development and validation of criterion-referenced clinically relevant fitness standards for maintaining physical independence in later years. Gerontologist 2012;53(2):255–67.

36. Hernandez D, Rose DJ. Predicting which older adults will or will not fall using the fullerton advanced balance scale. Arch Phys Med Rehabil 2008;89:2309–15.

37. Mihaljcic T, Haines TP, Ponsford JL, et al. Investigating the relationship between reduced self-awareness of falls risk, rehabilitation engagement and falls in older adults. Arch Gerontol Geriatr 2017;69:18–44.

38. Rose DJ. Balance efficacy scale FallProof!™: a comprehensive balance and mobility training program. 2nd edition. Champaign (IL): Human Kinetics; 2010. p. 80–1, 104–106.

39. Laidlaw K, Kishita N, Shenkin SD, et al. Development of a short form of the attitudes to aging Questionnaire (AAQ). Int J Geriatr Psychiatry 2018;33:113–21.

40. Hausdorf JM, Levy BR, Wei JY. The power of ageism on physical function of older persons: reversibility of age-related gait changes. J Am Geriatr Soc 1999;47:1346–9.

41. Avaialble at: https://www.cdc.gov/steadi/pdf/STEADI-Brochure-StayIndependent-508.pdf. Accessed November 1, 2018.

42. Verghese J, Holtzer R, Lipton RB, et al. Quantitative gait markers and incident fall risk in older adults. J Gerontol A Biol Sci Med Sci 2009;64A(8):896–901.

43. Avaialble at: https://www.cdc.gov/steadi/pdf/STEADI-Assessment-4Stage-508.pdf. Accessed November 1, 2018.

44. Rose DJ, Jones J, Lucchese N. Predicting the probability of falls in community-residing older adults using the 8-ft up and go: a new measure of functional mobility. J Aging Phys Act 2002;10:466–75.

45. Avaialble at: https://www.cdc.gov/steadi/pdf/STEADI-Assessment-TUG-508.pdf
46. Zhang F, Ferrucci L, Culham E, et al. Performance on five times sit-to-stand task as a predictor of subsequent falls and disability in older persons. J Aging Health 2013;25(3):478–92.
47. Avaialble at: https://www.cdc.gov/steadi/pdf/STEADI-Assessment-30Sec-508.pdf. Accessed November 1, 2018.
48. Purser JL, Weinberger M, Cohen HJ, et al. Walking speed predicts health status and hospital costs for frail elderly male veterans. J Rehabil Res Dev 2005;42(4): 535–46.

Falls, Footwear, and Podiatric Interventions in Older Adults

Anna Lucy Hatton, PhD[a],*, Keith Rome, PhD, MSc[b]

KEYWORDS

- Footwear • Shoe insoles • Falls • Balance • Gait • Podiatry • Older adults

KEY POINTS

- Ill-fitting footwear and suboptimal footwear design can lead to foot and balance problems in older adults, which are modifiable behavioral risk factors for falls.
- Comfort is one key factor influencing footwear selection in older adults, many of whom choose to wear slippers indoors, which can increase falls risk.
- For older adults with diabetes and inflammatory arthritis, footwear interventions can help prevent ulcers and relieve pain; however, their effects on balance remain unclear.
- Footwear devices designed to provide sensory cues at the feet, may help improve balance and walking and reduce falls in older adults with neurodegenerative disease.
- Multifaceted podiatric interventions, which provide older adults with appropriate footwear, foot orthoses, and footwear education, are emerging as a strategy to help prevent falls.

INTRODUCTION

One in 3 community-dwelling adults older than 65 years will fall at least once each year.[1] Age-related foot problems, including foot pain caused by local factors (ie, structural disorders affecting the load-bearing bones of the foot) and systemic factors (ie, dermatologic, vascular, neurologic, and musculoskeletal conditions), are associated with falls in older adults.[2–5] Therefore, multifaceted podiatric interventions, including appropriate footwear, is a rapidly growing area of clinical practice to help prevent falls.[6–9]

Footwear is constantly developing to provide protection, accommodate deformities, and assist in the biomechanical function of the foot, ankle, and lower limb.[10] Footwear can also play a pivotal role in postural stability by enhancing plantar

Disclosure Statement: The authors have nothing to disclose.
a School of Health and Rehabilitation Sciences, University of Queensland, Therapies Building (84A), St Lucia, Brisbane, Queensland 4072, Australia; b School of Clinical Sciences, Auckland University of Technology, 90 Akoranga Drive, AA Building, Northcote, Auckland 0627, New Zealand
* Corresponding author.
E-mail address: a.hatton1@uq.edu.au

somatosensory feedback[11] or controlling foot motion.[12,13] Previous work in older adults has reported that poor footwear and design features, such as elevated heels, soft soles, and slip-on styles, can lead to postural instability, associated with falls.[14–16] This review summarizes the relationship between footwear designs and falls in older adults; considers footwear and falls in aging populations with metabolic disease, inflammatory arthritis, and neurodegenerative disease; and highlights the role of podiatric interventions (eg, footwear, foot orthoses, and patient education) in falls prevention strategies for older adults.

FOOTWEAR DESIGN AND FALLS

The association between footwear and falls is commonly attributed to suboptimal design features, including outer soles with tread patterns that offer limited or excessive traction with the supporting surface,[17] destabilizing heel dimensions (elevated/narrow heel),[14] and inadequate or absent fastenings that allow slip of the shoe on the foot.[18] A case-control study by Keegan and colleagues[19] examined the characteristics of adults who sustained falls-related fractures to the upper arm, forearm, pelvis, or lower limb, relative to those who fell but did not fracture. Of the 2348 falls reported, wearing shoes with a medium-/high-width or narrow-width heel was associated with an increased risk of fracture. Laboratory-based assessments suggest that an elevated heel may heighten the risk of falls,[20] due to deleterious effects on balance control[14,15] and underlying changes in lower limb muscle mechanics.[21,22] In comparison, another study reported that of 95 older fallers, only 2% were wearing high-heeled shoes at the time of sustaining a fall-related hip fracture, and other styles of footwear, specifically slippers (22%), walking boots (17%), and sandals (8%), were more commonly worn at the time of fall.[23] This discrepancy in findings[19,23] could be due to differences in footwear selection across the life span. High-heeled shoes may be less frequently worn with increasing age, possibly as a result of effective falls prevention strategies recommending "safe" footwear[24] or alternatively choosing shoes for their therapeutic benefit (eg, pain relief) rather than aesthetic value.[25]

Shoes comprising a basic construct rubber sole with a soft canvas upper (eg, athletic shoes) have been suggested to pose the lowest risk of falls in older adults.[26] Relative to athletic shoes, all other footwear styles (including lace-up oxfords, loafers, flats, boots, high heels, sandals, slippers) increase the likelihood of falling, with unshod conditions, such as barefoot or wearing socks with no shoes, being most strongly associated with slips and falls.[26] Although nonslip socks (comprising rubber grip components) appear to optimize gait patterns and minimize slip propensity in older adults, compared with wearing standard socks[27] or backless slippers,[28] they may not offer comparable benefits to that of appropriate footwear with regard to fall and injury prevention.[29] A review by Hartung and Lalonde[29] concluded that although nonslip socks are commonly used in hospitals as a temporary footwear solution for older patients, they can pose 2 major safety hazards. First, there is conflicting evidence concerning the potential for nonslip socks to help prevent falls, and second, wearing nonslip socks may heighten the risk of spreading infection in hospitalized older patients.[29] This evidence further challenges the use of nonslip socks (particularly within clinical settings), and supports the notion for older adults to rather wear their own appropriate, safe footwear.

FOOTWEAR FIT AND SELECTION

Ill-fitting shoes are a major precursor to falls, therefore an understanding of the aging foot, including older adults' footwear preferences, is paramount to achieve falls prevention. Foot problems in older adults commonly include deformities affecting the greater (eg, bunions) or lesser toes, edema, or changes in foot posture (eg, flatfeet), which alter foot morphology.[30] Gender differences exist in foot anthropometric measures, specifically toe height, toe angle, heel angle, and medial ball length.[30] In women, the feet are reported to widen at the forefoot between the ages of 20 to 80 years,[31] signified by larger measures of width and circumference at the ball of the foot, high instep, and heel instep.[31] Up to 90% of older adults also present with hyperkeratotic lesions (eg, corns, calluses), which are commonly exacerbated by changes in foot shape or wearing ill-fitting shoes, and if left untreated pose a high risk of falls, due to complications such as pain and ulcers.[4] In a prospective study of footwear preferences in 100 older adults,[32] only 5 people with hyperkeratotic lesions and 9 people without hyperkeratotic lesions reported wearing optimal shoes, characterized as "lace-ups, with extra width across the metatarsal heads, extra depth in the toe box, low heels, and a padded tongue." This evidence reinforces the need for continual review of footwear fit to accommodate structural changes and accompanying symptoms (eg, pain, calluses) in the aging foot (**Fig. 1**).

Perceived comfort is one of the primary criteria influencing older adults' choice of footwear,[25] yet may come at a cost to safety. Slippers are an attractive indoor footwear option for older adults, as they are convenient and comfortable, owing to their ease of wear (eg, slip-on style) and thick soft midsoles, yet these same features, in addition to smooth outer soles that offer minimal traction, can also heighten the risk of falls.[33,34] A survey of 128 community-dwelling older Australians reported that slippers were the most commonly worn style of household footwear, whereas more than one-quarter of respondents preferred to go barefoot or wear socks without shoes.[35] This preference for slippers or to remain unshod is of serious concern. The MOBILZE Boston Study[34] reported that ~52% of 563 falls experienced in the home occurred when older adults were barefoot, or wearing socks (without shoes) or slippers. Furthermore, Menz and colleagues[36] evaluated standing balance and walking ability in 30 older women while wearing socks and 2 different styles of slippers. Enclosed slippers with a firm sole and secure fastening, were reported to optimize measures of balance (eg, postural sway, limits of stability) and gait (eg, spatiotemporal parameters), when compared with soft, backless slippers or socks without shoes. This evidence supports earlier work suggesting that footwear devices constructed from soft

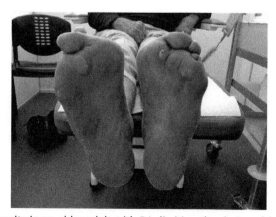

Fig. 1. Foot deformity in an older adult with RA, limiting the choice of footwear available that will accommodate altered foot shape.

material may dampen vital plantar sensory information, which is critical for balance.[11,15]

FOOTWEAR AND FALLS IN DISEASE POPULATIONS
Diabetes Mellitus

Falls are a major concern for older adults with diabetes mellitus, with annual incidence rates of 39% in those older than 65 years, increasing to 54% for those with previous foot ulceration.[37] Common risk factors for falls within this population include peripheral neuropathy, foot complications (eg, ulceration), impaired postural control, polypharmacy, suboptimal glycemic control, as well as vision and cognitive impairment.[38]

Foot care is standard practice in diabetes management, with therapeutic footwear and shoe insoles commonly issued to help prevent foot ulcers[39] or alleviate pain resulting from high plantar pressures. Few studies have explored the effect of traditional shoe insoles on postural control in adults with diabetic neuropathy, reporting inconclusive findings both supporting[40] and refuting[41] the efficacy of insoles. Offloading footwear is commonly recommended for foot ulcers, yet can have a negative effect on postural control.[42] A review by Buldt and Menz[43] also reported that older people with diabetes and current foot ulceration were up to 5 times more likely to be wearing ill-fitting shoes compared with individuals without foot ulceration.

From a patient's perspective, a qualitative study considered the footwear choices of people with diabetic neuropathy and a history of falls.[44] Although most participants did not believe that their footwear (worn at the time of fall) contributed to their fall, most did consider their footwear to influence their perceived balance confidence when completing daily activities. Most participants found their therapeutic footwear "difficult" to walk in, "heavy," or "slippery bottomed." Footwear design features, considered to enhance balance, included a close fit, tight fastening, lightweight, substantial tread, and a firm, moulded sole. Notably, hiking sandals were deemed to be a stable and safe choice of footwear, and most frequently worn to help reduce fear of falling and boost confidence during walking.[44]

For older adults with diabetic peripheral neuropathy, novel footwear devices (eg, textured or vibratory insoles) designed to provide substitute sensory cues at the feet, are emerging as an attractive treatment option to help ameliorate balance and gait deficits[45–47] (**Fig. 2**). Design modifications to offloading footwear, such as reduction in strut height and reduced weight, may also improve postural stability and reduce falls risk.[48]

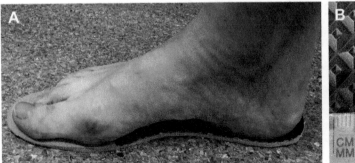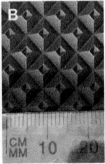

Fig. 2. Sensory stimulating insoles for diabetic peripheral neuropathy. (A) Poron base with polyvinyl chloride textured material extending from the heel to metatarsal heads. (B) Textured material comprising raised pyramidal nodules.

Inflammatory Arthritis

Foot-related studies concerning falls in inflammatory arthritis have predominantly focused on rheumatoid arthritis (RA): a chronic, autoimmune disease and the most common form of polyarticular arthritis. When first diagnosed, ~16% of people with RA may have foot involvement, increasing to 90% with longer disease duration.[49] Brenton-Rule and colleagues[50] reported that falls incidence ranged from 10% to 50% in people with RA. Swollen and tender lower extremity joints, pain intensity, and poor balance were among multiple factors identified to increase falls risk. In a cross-sectional study of adults with established RA, elevated midfoot peak plantar pressures and self-reported foot impairment were associated with falls in the preceding 12 months.[51] However, in a 12-month prospective study, foot and ankle characteristics were not associated with falls in people with RA, independent of prior falls.[52] Morpeth and colleagues[53] highlighted the important relationship between fear of falling, foot impairment, and disability, which warrants further consideration as a vital component of future clinical screening tools to assess falls risk.

There is little evidence regarding the impact of therapeutic footwear on impaired balance in people with RA. We do know that as RA progresses, localized forefoot deformities, such as hallux valgus and clawing of the lesser toes, occur, leading to a high proportion of people with RA wearing sandals,[54] or in some cases, self-modifying their footwear (**Fig. 3**). However, sandals offer limited motion control, and have been found to be detrimental to the standing balance of older women with established RA, particularly when visual information is limited (eg, eyes closed).[55]

Parkinson Disease

Annually, between 45% and 68% of older adults with Parkinson disease will experience at least 1 fall,[56,57] with up to two-thirds falling on multiple occasions.[58] Although several falls risk factors specific to people with Parkinson disease are nonremediable (eg, disease severity and duration), "freezing of gait" and "impaired balance" can be modified through physical interventions.[59] Although podiatry care is not routinely offered to adults with Parkinson disease, there has been an increase in the development of new footwear devices,[60,61] including laser shoes,[62] and vibratory[63] and textured[64–66] shoe insoles, designed to provide sensory cues at the feet to optimize balance and gait.

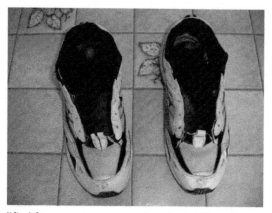

Fig. 3. Patient-modified footwear to accommodate foot deformities.

Laser shoes, which project an intermittent beam in front of an individual's contralateral foot,[67] can provide visual cues to help reduce freezing of gait in Parkinson disease, specifically the number of "freezing" episodes and time spent "frozen."[62] Vibratory shoe insoles that provide step-synchronized stimuli to the foot can also enhance spatiotemporal gait measures in people with Parkinson disease[63]; however, it is unclear whether such changes translate to a reduction in falls.

Textured shoe insoles also may have the capacity to ameliorate gait and balance deficits in Parkinson disease. Immediate effects of using a ribbed insole (relative to a flat insole) have included increased single-limb support time, in 40 adults with Parkinson disease.[65] Similarly, Lirani-Silva and colleagues[64] observed greater stride length in 10 adults with Parkinson disease following short-term wear (1-week) of textured insoles. However, improvements in gait parameters were not maintained at a subsequent 1-week follow-up, suggesting prolonged wear may be required to bring about long-term changes. Qiu and colleagues[66] reported that textured insoles have the capacity to reduce mediolateral sway during standing in people with Parkinson disease, when visual and somatosensory inputs are manipulated (eg, eyes closed, foam surface). This is a clinically relevant finding, as measures of mediolateral balance control are considered to be strong predictors of recurrent[68] and future[69] falls.

A recent survey explored the footwear habits, foot problems, and falls status of adults with Parkinson disease and stroke.[70] Of the 218 respondents with Parkinson disease, 50% reported falling at least once each year, and more than half (53%) experienced foot problems that impacted their balance and footwear selection. Comfort and fit were considered the most important factors underpinning shoe selection, often to accommodate foot problems.[70] However, of concern, slippers were the most common choice of indoor footwear by 35% of adults with Parkinson disease, yet pose a high risk of falls.[33,34] A large proportion of fallers (47%) were not receiving foot care,[70] highlighting the urgent need for greater awareness, development, and implementation of podiatry interventions for older adults with neurodegenerative disease.

FOOTWEAR IN MULTIFACTORIAL FALLS PREVENTION PROGRAMS

Footwear, insoles, and orthoses are gaining popularity as an integral component of falls prevention strategies.[6–9] A randomized clinical trial of 305 community-dwelling older adults with disabling foot pain in Australia explored the effects of a multifaceted podiatry intervention, comprising foot and ankle exercises, orthoses, a voucher to purchase new appropriate footwear (as required), and footwear and falls prevention advice, on the rate of falls.[8] Relative to usual podiatry care (eg, treatment for corns), participants in the intervention group reported 36% fewer falls in the 12 months following randomization.[8] A similar podiatry intervention was implemented in 1010 community-dwelling older adults (without foot pain) in the United Kingdom and Ireland.[6,7] All participants received routine podiatry care and a falls prevention leaflet, whereas the intervention group additionally received footwear advice, the provision of new footwear (where current footwear was deemed inappropriate), foot orthoses, and a home-based foot and ankle exercise program (with supporting DVD and booklet). The intervention group demonstrated a significantly lower proportion of older adults who experienced 1 or more falls.[6,7] However, satisfaction with the trial footwear was variable, with comfort and shoe-sizing emerging as critical factors underlying adherence. For older adults living in nursing homes, evidence suggests that multifaceted podiatry interventions are also feasible to implement within this setting: further evaluation of their capacity to reduce falls is required.[9]

FUTURE DIRECTIONS

Footwear is a modifiable falls risk factor in older adults showing age-related degeneration and for those with disease-specific symptoms. An ideal safe shoe, which can enhance balance and gait, and reduce falls is not yet commercially available. Design recommendations for such a shoe include a low broad heel, thin firm midsole, high collar, and slip-resistant outer sole.[71,72] On this basis, prototype footwear[73] and novel shoe insoles[45] for older adults are emerging, and show promise in their acceptability to users, capacity to improve balance and mobility, and reduce falls. Importantly, emerging evidence suggests that podiatric interventions, when accompanied by foot health and footwear education, may play a vital role in multifaceted falls prevention strategies.

SUMMARY

This review has demonstrated that ill-fitting footwear, and specific footwear design features, can impair balance control and heighten the risk of falling in older adults. Although foot care is routine practice for some older adults to prevent foot ulceration in high-risk populations, such as those with diabetes, or reduce foot pain, impairment and disability in people with inflammatory arthritis, new footwear interventions are emerging with the potential to enhance balance and mobility. Multifaceted podiatric interventions, which include appropriate footwear and importantly patient education, may also have the capacity to help reduce falls in older adults.

REFERENCES

1. Tinetti ME, Speechley M, Ginter SF. Risk factors for falls among elderly persons living in the community. N Engl J Med 1988;319:1701–7.
2. Awale A, Hagedorn TJ, Dufour AB, et al. Foot function, foot pain, and falls in older adults: the Framingham foot study. Gerontology 2017;63:318–24.
3. Menz HB. Chronic foot pain in older people. Maturitas 2016;91:110–4.
4. Menz HB, Morris ME, Lord SR. Foot and ankle risk factors for falls in older people: a prospective study. J Gerontol A Biol Sci Med Sci 2006;61:866–70.
5. Mickle KJ, Munro BJ, Lord SR, et al. Foot pain, plantar pressures, and falls in older people: a prospective study. J Am Geriatr Soc 2010;58:1936–40.
6. Cockayne S, Adamson J, Clarke A, et al. Cohort randomised controlled trial of a multifaceted podiatry intervention for the prevention of falls in older people (The REFORM Trial). PLoS One 2017;12(1):e0168712.
7. Corbacho B, Cockayne S, Fairhurst C, et al. Cost-effectiveness of a multifaceted podiatry intervention for the prevention of falls in older people: the REducing Falls with orthoses and a multifaceted podiatry intervention trial findings. Gerontology 2018;26:1–10.
8. Spink MJ, Menz HB, Fotoohabadi MR, et al. Effectiveness of a multifaceted podiatry intervention to prevent falls in community dwelling older people with disabling foot pain: randomised controlled trial. BMJ 2011;342:d3411.
9. Wylie G, Menz HB, McFarlane S, et al. Podiatry intervention versus usual care to prevent falls in care homes: pilot randomised controlled trial (the PIRFECT study). BMC Geriatr 2017;17:143.
10. Williams AE, Nester CJ. Patient perception of stock footwear design features. Prosthet Orthot Int 2006;30:61–71.

11. Perry SD, Radtke A, Goodwin CR. Influence of footwear midsole material hardness on dynamic balance control during unexpected gait termination. Gait Posture 2007;25(1):94–8.
12. Barton CJ, Bonanno D, Menz HB. Development and evaluation of a tool for the assessment of footwear characteristics. J Foot Ankle Res 2009;2:10.
13. Menz HB, Lord SR. Footwear and postural stability in older people. J Am Podiatr Med Assoc 1999;89:346–57.
14. Lord SR, Bashford GM. Shoe characteristics and balance in older women. J Am Geriatr Soc 1996;44(4):429–33.
15. Menant JC, Perry SD, Steele JR, et al. Effects of shoe characteristics on dynamic stability when walking on even and uneven surfaces in young and older people. Arch Phys Med Rehabil 2008;89(10):1970–6.
16. Menant JC, Steele JR, Menz HB, et al. Effects of footwear features on balance and stepping in older people. Gerontology 2008;54:18–23.
17. Connell BR, Wolf SL. Environmental and behavioral circumstances associated with falls at home among healthy elderly individuals. Atlanta FICSIT Group. Arch Phys Med Rehabil 1997;78(2):179–86.
18. Gabell A, Simons MA, Nayak US. Falls in the healthy elderly: predisposing causes. Ergonomics 1985;28(7):965–75.
19. Keegan TH, Kelsey JL, King AC, et al. Characteristics of fallers who fracture at the foot, distal forearm, proximal humerus, pelvis, and shaft of the tibia/fibula compared with fallers who do not fracture. Am J Epidemiol 2004;159(2):192–203.
20. Tencer AF, Koepsell TD, Wolf ME, et al. Biomechanical properties of shoes and risk of falls in older adults. J Am Geriatr Soc 2004;52(11):1840–6.
21. Cronin NJ, Barrett RS, Carty CP. Long-term use of high-heeled shoes alters the neuromechanics of human walking. J Appl Physiol 2012;112(6):1054–8.
22. Csapo R, Maganaris CN, Seynnes OR, et al. On muscle, tendon and high heels. J Exp Biol 2010;213:2582–8.
23. Sherrington C, Menz HB. An evaluation of footwear worn at the time of fall-related hip fracture. Age Ageing 2003;32(3):310–4.
24. Kempton A, van Beurden E, Sladden T, et al. Older people can stay on their feet: final results of a community-based falls prevention programme. Health Promot Int 2000;15(1):27–33.
25. Davis A, Murphy A, Haines TP. "Good for older ladies, not me": how elderly women choose their shoes. J Am Podiatr Med Assoc 2013;103(6):465–70.
26. Koepsell TD, Wolf ME, Buchner DM, et al. Footwear style and risk of falls in older adults. J Am Geriatr Soc 2004;52(9):1495–501.
27. Hatton AL, Sturnieks DL, Lord SR, et al. Effects of nonslip socks on the gait patterns of older people when walking on a slippery surface. J Am Podiatr Med Assoc 2013;103(6):471–9.
28. Hübscher M, Thiel C, Schmidt J, et al. Slip resistance of non-slip socks—an accelerometer-based approach. Gait Posture 2011;33(4):740–52.
29. Hartung B, Lalonde M. The use of non-slip socks to prevent falls among hospitalized older adults: a literature review. Geriatr Nurs 2017;38(5):412–6.
30. Mickle KJ, Munro BJ, Lord SR, et al. Foot shape of older people: implications for shoe design. Footwear Sci 2010;2(3):131–9.
31. Ansuategui Echeita J, Hijmans JM, Smits S, et al. Age-related differences in women's foot shape. Maturitas 2016;94:64–9.
32. Palomo-López P, Becerro-de-Bengoa-Vallejo R, Losa-Iglesias ME, et al. Footwear used by older people and a history of hyperkeratotic lesions on the foot: a prospective observational study. Medicine 2017;96(15):e6623.

33. Kerse N, Butler M, Robinson E, et al. Wearing slippers, falls and injury in residential care. Aust N Z J Public Health 2004;28(2):180–7.
34. Kelsey JL, Procter-Gray E, Nguyen US, et al. Footwear and falls in the home among older individuals in the MOBILIZE Boston study. Footwear Sci 2010; 2(3):123–9.
35. Munro BJ, Steele JR. Household-shoe wearing and purchasing habits. A survey of people aged 65 years and older. J Am Podiatr Med Assoc 1999;89(10): 506–14.
36. Menz HB, Auhl M, Munteanu SE. Effects of indoor footwear on balance and gait patterns in community-dwelling older women. Gerontology 2017;63(2):129–36.
37. Macgilchrist C, Paul L, Ellis BM, et al. Lower-limb risk factors for falls in people with diabetes mellitus. Diabet Med 2010;27:162–8.
38. Chapman A, Meyer C. Falls prevention in older adults with diabetes: a clinical review of screening, assessment and management recommendations. Diabetes Primary Care Australia 2017;2:69–74.
39. Lavery LA, LaFontaine J, Higgins KR, et al. Shear-reducing insoles to prevent foot ulceration in high-risk diabetic patients. Adv Skin Wound Care 2012;25:519–24.
40. Ites KI, Anderson EJ, Cahill ML, et al. Balance interventions for diabetic peripheral neuropathy: a systematic review. J Geriatr Phys Ther 2011;34:109–16.
41. Van Geffen JA, Dijkstra PU, Hof AL, et al. Effect of flat insoles with different Shore A values on posture stability in diabetic neuropathy. Prosthet Orthot Int 2007;31: 228–35.
42. Van Deursen R. Footwear for the neuropathic patient: offloading and stability. Diabetes Metab Res Rev 2008;24:S96–100.
43. Buldt AK, Menz HB. Incorrectly fitted footwear, foot pain and foot disorders: a systematic search and narrative review of the literature. J Foot Ankle Res 2018;11:43.
44. Paton JS, Roberts A, Bruce GK, et al. Does footwear affect balance? The views and experiences of people with diabetes and neuropathy who have fallen. J Am Podiatr Med Assoc 2013;103(6):508–15.
45. Hatton AL, Dixon J, Rome K, et al. Altering gait by way of stimulation of the plantar surface of the foot: the immediate effect of wearing textured insoles in older fallers. J Foot Ankle Res 2012;5:11.
46. Hijmans JM, Geertzen JH, Zijlstra W, et al. Effects of vibrating insoles on standing balance in diabetic neuropathy. J Rehabil Res Dev 2008;45(9):1441–9.
47. Lipsitz LA, Lough M, Niemi J, et al. A shoe insole delivering subsensory vibratory noise improves balance and gait in healthy elderly people. Arch Phys Med Rehabil 2015;96(3):432–9.
48. Crews RT, Sayeed F, Najafi B. Impact of strut height on offloading capacity of removable cast walkers. Clin Biomech 2012;27:725–30.
49. Otter SJ, Lucas K, Springett K, et al. Foot pain in rheumatoid arthritis prevalence, risk factors and management: an epidemiological study. Clin Rheumatol 2010;29: 255–71.
50. Brenton-Rule A, Dalbeth N, Bassett S, et al. The incidence and risk factors for falls in adults with rheumatoid arthritis: a systematic review. Semin Arthritis Rheum 2015;44:389–98.
51. Brenton-Rule A, Dalbeth N, Menz HB, et al. Foot and ankle characteristics associated with falls in adults with established rheumatoid arthritis: a cross-sectional study. BMC Musculoskelet Disord 2016;17:22.
52. Brenton-Rule A, Dallbeth N, Menz HB, et al. Are foot and ankle characteristics associated with falls in people with rheumatoid arthritis? A prospective study. Arthritis Care Res 2017;69:1150–5.

53. Morpeth T, Brenton-Rule A, Carroll M, et al. Fear of falling and foot pain, impairment and disability in rheumatoid arthritis: a case-control study. Clin Rheumatol 2016;35:887–91.

54. Brenton-Rule A, Hendry GJ, Barr G, et al. An evaluation of seasonal variations in footwear worn by adults with inflammatory arthritis: a cross-sectional observational study using a web-based survey. J Foot Ankle Res 2014;7:36.

55. Brenton-Rule A, D'Almeida S, Bassett S, et al. The effects of sandals on postural stability in patients with rheumatoid arthritis: an exploratory study. Clin Biomech 2014;29:350–3.

56. Latt MD, Lord SR, Morris JG, et al. Clinical and physiological assessments for elucidating falls risk in Parkinson's disease. Mov Disord 2009;24(9):1280–9.

57. Wood BH, Bilclough JA, Bowron A, et al. Incidence and prediction of falls in Parkinson's disease: a prospective multidisciplinary study. J Neurol Neurosurg Psychiatry 2002;72(6):721–5.

58. Allen NE, Schwarzel AK, Canning CG. Recurrent falls in Parkinson's disease: a systematic review. Parkinsons Dis 2013;2013:906274.

59. Canning CG, Paul SS, Nieuwboer A. Prevention of falls in Parkinson's disease: a review of fall risk factors and the role of physical interventions. Neurodegener Dis Manag 2014;4(3):203–21.

60. Maculewicz J, Kofoed LB, Serafin S. A technological review of the instrumented footwear for rehabilitation with a focus on Parkinson's disease patients. Front Neurol 2016;7:1.

61. Alfuth M. Textured and stimulating insoles for balance and gait impairments in patients with multiple sclerosis and Parkinson's disease: a systematic review and meta-analysis. Gait Posture 2017;51:132–41.

62. Barthel C, Nonnekes J, van Helvert M, et al. The laser shoes: a new ambulatory device to alleviate freezing of gait in Parkinson disease. Neurology 2018;90(2): e164–71.

63. Novak P, Novak V. Effect of step-synchronized vibration stimulation of soles on gait in Parkinson's disease: a pilot study. J Neuroeng Rehabil 2006;3:9.

64. Lirani-Silva E, Vitório R, Barbieri FA, et al. Continuous use of textured insole improve plantar sensation and stride length of people with Parkinson's disease: a pilot study. Gait Posture 2017;58:495–7.

65. Jenkins ME, Almeida QJ, Spaulding SJ, et al. Plantar cutaneous sensory stimulation improves single-limb support time, and EMG activation patterns among individuals with Parkinson's disease. Parkinsonism Relat Disord 2009;15(9):697–702.

66. Qiu F, Cole MH, Davids KW, et al. Effects of textured insoles on balance in people with Parkinson's disease. PLoS One 2013;8(12):e83309.

67. Ferraye MU, Fraix V, Pollak P, et al. The laser-shoe: a new form of continuous ambulatory cueing for patients with Parkinson's disease. Parkinsonism Relat Disord 2016;29:127–8.

68. Stel V, Smit J, Pluijm S, et al. Balance and mobility performance as treatable risk factors for recurrent falling in older persons. J Clin Epidemiol 2003;56:659–68.

69. Maki B, Holliday P, Topper A. A prospective study of postural balance and risk of falling in an ambulatory and independent elderly population. J Gerontol A Biol Sci Med Sci 1994;49:M72–84.

70. Bowen C, Ashburn A, Cole M, et al. A survey exploring self-reported indoor and outdoor footwear habits, foot problems and fall status in people with stroke and Parkinson's. J Foot Ankle Res 2016;9(1):39.

71. Aboutorabi A, Bahramizadeh M, Arazpour M, et al. A systematic review of the effect of foot orthoses and shoe characteristics on balance in healthy older subjects. Prosthet Orthot Int 2016;40:170–81.
72. Menant JC, Steele JR, Menz HB, et al. Optimizing footwear for older people at risk of falls. J Rehabil Res Dev 2008;45(8):1167–81.
73. Menz HB, Auhl M, Munteanu SE. Preliminary evaluation of prototype footwear and insoles to optimise balance and gait in older people. BMC Geriatr 2017;17:212.

Balance Problems and Fall Risks in the Elderly

Ramon Cuevas-Trisan, MD

KEYWORDS

- Balance • Falls • Older adults • Risk factors

KEY POINTS

- Fall prevention strategies are important interventions in all elderly individuals.
- Prevention of falls can decrease morbidity and mortality in the elderly.
- Evaluation and effective intervention strategies are generally multifactorial.

INTRODUCTION
Demographics and Scope of the Problem

Falls are an important cause of morbidity and mortality and the leading cause of fatal and nonfatal injuries among older adults. According to data obtained from the Behavioral Risk Factor Surveillance System survey and analyzed by the Centers for Disease Control and Prevention, in 2014, approximately 28.7% of older adults reported falling at least once in the preceding 12 months, resulting in an estimated 29.0 million falls and 7.0 million fall injuries in the United States.[1] Injury severity varies but 2.8 million were treated in emergency departments for fall-related injuries and approximately 800,000 of these individuals were subsequently hospitalized. Of those who fell, 37.5% reported at least one fall that required medical treatment or restricted activity for at least 1 day.[1] Approximately 27,000 older adults died because of falls during that same period.

Women are more likely to report falling and to report a fall injury than men. The percentage of older adults who fall increases with age, from 26.7% among persons aged 65 to 74 years, to 29.8% among persons aged 75 to 84 years, to 36.5% among persons aged greater than or equal to 85 years.[2] It is generally known that falling in the elderly is usually caused by various factors. Therefore, multifactorial interventions may be more effective than any one single intervention.

This article originally appeared in *Physical Medicine and Rehabilitation Clinics of North America*, Volume 28, Issue 4, November 2017.
Disclosures: The author has nothing to disclose.
Physical Medicine and Rehabilitation Service, West Palm Beach VA Medical Center, University of Miami Miller School of Medicine, Nova Southeastern University College of Osteopathic Medicine, 7305 North Military Trail, PM&RS (117), West Palm Beach, FL 33410-6400, USA
E-mail address: ramon.cuevas-trisan@va.gov

Clin Geriatr Med 35 (2019) 173–183
https://doi.org/10.1016/j.cger.2019.01.008

PATIENT ASSESSMENT
Conditions

Gait and balance disorders

Gait and balance disorders are among the most common causes of falls in older adults and often lead to injury, disability, loss of independence, and limitations in quality of life. Good balance is likely a rapid synergistic interaction between various physiologic and cognitive elements that allow rapid and precise response to a perturbation.[3] It is a remarkably complex relationship between systems that allow for rapid and precise changes to prevent a fall (concept of reaction time). Gait and balance disorders are usually multifactorial in origin and require a comprehensive assessment to determine contributing factors and targeted interventions. Most changes in gait occurring in older adults are related to underlying medical conditions, particularly as conditions increase in severity, and should not be viewed as merely an inevitable consequence of aging. Early identification of gait and balance disorders and appropriate intervention may prevent dysfunction and loss of independence.[4] The prevalence of abnormal gait increases with age and is higher in persons in the acute hospital setting and in those living in long-term care facilities.

Cognitive impairment

Neurocognitive functions powerfully influence fall risk.[5] Cognitive impairment, regardless of the diagnosis, is a risk factor for falls.[6] Cognitively impaired adults show an increased risk of falls compared with their age-matched cognitively intact peers.[7] The increasing incidence of various forms of dementia and degrees of cognitive impairment in older adults has increased the prevalence of falls in this population.[8]

Early fall prevention in adults with mild cognitive problems follows a strong rationale. This population is at high risk of functional decline and generally has significant comorbidities. Falls can contribute to this decline through injury, hospital admission, loss of confidence, and deconditioning from reduced activity. Any intervention that can reduce the risk of future falls at an early stage has the potential to maintain function and activity level, thus reducing the progression into disability and dependency. By helping people to adopt techniques to stay healthy (ie, strength and balance exercises) and adaptations that reduce risk (ie, appropriate mobility aids, home hazard reduction) at an early stage of cognitive impairment, these practices could theoretically help as cognitive decline progresses.[8] Cognitive assessment is strongly advised but there is no clear guidance on how to respond to individuals with cognitive impairment because recommendations and evidence for effective fall prevention interventions for older adults with cognitive impairment are not well documented.[9]

Musculoskeletal conditions and pain

Persistent pain, impaired mobility and function, and reduced quality of life are the most common experiences associated with musculoskeletal conditions. The prevalence and impact of musculoskeletal conditions increase with aging. Population growth, aging, and sedentary lifestyles, particularly in developing countries, have created a crisis for population health that requires a multisystem response with musculoskeletal health services as a critical component. Globally, there is an emphasis on maintaining an active lifestyle to fight numerous ailments associated with sedentary habits. However, painful musculoskeletal conditions profoundly limit the ability of people to make these lifestyle changes. A strong relationship exists between painful musculoskeletal conditions and a reduced capacity to engage in physical activity resulting in functional decline, frailty, reduced well-being, and loss of independence. In a group of community-dwelling adults older than 88 years in the Netherlands, joint pain was reported as the most common contributor to gait problems, followed by several other causes.[10] The use of mobility aids (eg, various types of canes and walkers) can help with stability and help reduce the contribution of musculoskeletal problems to falls. These, however, must be properly adjusted or fitted for the individual to effectively help unload painful joints. Additionally, when improperly prescribed, these could result in the patients not using them or worse yet, contribute to increase the incidence of falls.[11] Many physiatric therapies and interventions are available to address the negative impact of musculoskeletal conditions.

Vision

Visual impairment is an underrepresented area of research for falls among older adults but is generally recognized to be an important risk factor. The prevalence of vision impairment and blindness increases with age and poor vision as a risk factor for falls is sometimes overlooked because the process of decreasing vision is often slow and may even be unnoticeable for some older individuals. Impaired visual acuity increases the risk of falls and injuries, and bilateral visual field loss caused by glaucoma is associated with greater fear of falling with an impact that exceeds numerous other risk factors.[12]

Improving visual function may have benefits, such as decreased traumatic events and improved mobility. However, changes should be made with caution because well-meaning and rational interventions can increase the risk of falls (a study found that the falling rate of the visually intervened was higher than in the control group).[13] One possible explanation is that improved vision may lead to changes in behavior that increase exposure to fall-pone situations. Additionally, vision-related interventions tend to focus on correcting central vision when both central and peripheral vision components may be necessary to effectively reduce rates of falls.[12] Investigators analyzed data from seven high-quality studies evaluating visual problems as risk factors targeting interventions for visual loss. They identified various combinations of targeted interventions in the setting of visual impairment and concluded that visual intervention plus various risk factor assessments and interventions were more effective than visual intervention alone or other combined interventions (eg, exercise and vision) in preventing falls in older people.[12] A Cochrane review on the subject also revealed that first eye cataract surgery reduces the rate of falls.[11]

Medications

The use of multiple medications (four or more), and specific classes of medications, can lead to gait and balance disorders and increased rate of falls.[14,15] The concept of medication reconciliation (the process of reviewing all the medications that a patient is taking prescribed by any and all providers) has gained importance and is increasingly being used in all clinical settings. It has long been recognized that polypharmacy is a source of many iatrogenic problems, from side effects caused by drug-drug interactions to continuation of unnecessary medications. Providers need to recognize that many medications, especially those with central nervous system effects, need to be used with caution in elderly individuals because of the effects that these could have altering their reaction time, memory, balance, and brain perfusion. Notable offenders include opioids, benzodiazepines, diuretics, vasodilators, tricyclic antidepressants, skeletal muscle relaxants, β-blockers, antihistamine medications, and sleep aids. Antiplatelet agents and anticoagulants, common in the elderly because of associated cardiovascular ailments, add another layer of complexity, potentially making falls catastrophic.

The practice of managing medication side effects with other medications, although common in the clinical setting, is rarely justified and physicians should always consider discontinuing and replacing the original medication before adding another to treat undesirable side effects.

Sarcopenia

Sarcopenia is a syndrome characterized by progressive and generalized loss of skeletal muscle mass and strength with a risk of adverse outcomes, such as physical disability, poor quality of life, and death.[16] Its precise diagnostic criteria and pathophysiology are beyond the scope of this article but its prevalence, which may be 30% for those older than 60 years of age, will increase as the percentage of the very old continues to grow.[17] Sarcopenia and physical frailty run along the same continuum. Physical frailty in its initial phase can still be reversed and fighting sarcopenia in elderly persons has the potential to slow or halt the progressive decline toward disability and dependency.

Box 1 provides an overview of potential causes for falls in older adults. The clinician should consider assessing for fall risk when any of these conditions are present.

Patient Evaluation

History

The patient's history should include specific questions about known risk factors for falls. It is imperative to ask about prior falls and the circumstances surrounding these, because patients who have fallen in the last year are significantly more likely to fall again (likelihood ratio, 2.3–2.8).[18]

The clinician should always inquire about environmental hazards. Some common hazards include poor lighting, rugs, areas of high clutter, electrical cords, slippery surfaces, steps, and stairways. Whenever possible, the clinician should include other family members in this conversation because patients tend to downplay the importance of some of these hazards. A functional history should always be obtained including ability to perform basic and instrumental activities of daily living.[4]

Physical examination

Inspection for joint deformities, swelling, and bruises is an important component of the examination. Joint instability and passive and active range of motion limitations in the major joints of the lower limb joints and spine should be evaluated, including assessing for soft tissue tightness that may produce limitations. Commonly encountered problems include tight hamstrings and tight iliopsoas, limiting knee and hip extension, respectively. These limitations alter the normal gait pattern and in turn the body's center of gravity, contributing to greater energy consumption during the gait cycle and balance challenges.

Posture, particularly excess kyphosis commonly seen in older persons, can significantly shift the body's center of gravity. Forward shift of the head with limited neck extension also alters the center of gravity and contributes to postural imbalance and limits the functional peripheral visual field.

Ideal footwear should fit properly, be comfortable (taking into account common foot deformities, such as hallux valgus and per cavus), provide wide support and stability, and be lightweight for ease during foot advancement.

A focused neurologic examination to detect deficits, such as sensory impairments (particularly proprioception), and weakness should always be performed because it may reveal potentially treatable problems. Proprioceptive impairment caused by a neuropathy, for example, is a common cause of balance impairment in older adults. Decreased vibration sense, a frequent but abnormal finding in this population, is a more sensitive marker of neuropathy than a decrease in position sense. Balance

---

Box 1
Risk factors associated with gait and balance disorders in the older adult

Neurologic disorders

Delirium/dementia

Cerebellar dysfunction

Myelopathy

Normal pressure hydrocephalus

Stroke

Parkinson's disease and related disorders

Peripheral neuropathies

Visual impairment

Myopathies

Cardiovascular disorders

Congestive heart failure

Arrhythmias

Peripheral arterial disease

Orthostatic hypotension

Musculoskeletal disorders

Spinal stenosis

Painful arthritides/spondylosis

Lower limb deformities

Muscle weakness and atrophy (sarcopenia)

Other medical disorders

Most acute medical illnesses

Medications: diuretics, opioids, benzodiazepines, anticonvulsants, antidepressants, psychotropics, anticholinergics, sleep aids

Obesity

Vitamin B_{12} deficiency

Diabetes

Uremia

Hepatic encephalopathy

Substance use disorders

This list is not comprehensive, but provides an overview of potential causes. The clinician should consider assessing for fall risk when any of these conditions are present.

---

that worsens with the eyes closed and improves when minor support is given by the examiner is another clue for proprioceptive problems.[19] Additionally, the clinician should assess for coordination, tone, tremors, cognition, and depression (usually with a validated questionnaire).

Evaluation of gait is an essential step to identify persons at fall risk. Observational gait assessment should assess velocity, stride length, antalgic movements, balance, stance, and symmetry. If it seems normal and functional, challenges should be introduced by asking the individual to walk on toes and heels. Tandem and backward walking, and unipedal stance, are particularly useful tests for detection of more subtle balance problems. These should be performed carefully and the clinician should be prepared to provide physical assistance if needed during testing to prevent a fall.

Observational ability to get up from a chair is also an excellent screening for function, testing proximal strength, balance, and coordination simultaneously. Other formal functional tests, such as the Timed Up and Go Test, are reliable and easy to administer. Such tests as the Berg Balance Scale and the Performance-Oriented Mobility Assessment are excellent but more time consuming. The Functional Reach Test is another reliable, valid, and quick diagnostic test for postural stability.[4] The general evaluation is not complete without obtaining the vital signs with particular attention to possible orthostatic hypotension, along with screenings for hearing and visual problems. Cardiovascular conditions are highly prevalent in older adults. Certain arrhythmias can lead to syncope and falls. A Cochrane database review concluded that pacemakers reduced the rate of falls in people with carotid sinus hypersensitivity.[11] When assessed appropriately, clinically significant postural hypotension is detected in up to 30% of elderly persons but unfortunately, some elderly persons with postural hypotension do not report symptoms, such as dizziness or lightheadedness.[19] **Fig. 1** provides an outline of the key components of the physical examination for an older adult at risk for falls. **Table 1** provides symptoms and signs and associated selected disorders causing decreased balance and falls in the older adult.

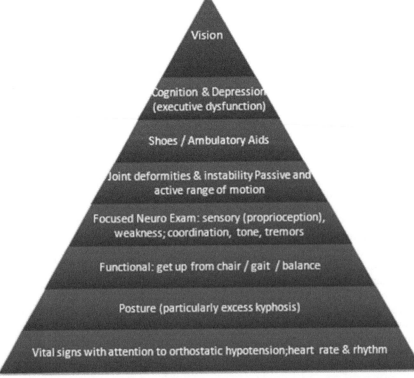

Fig. 1. Key physical examination components when evaluating an older adult for risk of falling.

Table 1
Symptoms and signs and associated disorders affecting gait/balance

Signs/Symptoms	Associated Disorders
Back pain, claudication (worsens with extension improved with flexion)	Spinal stenosis
Hyperreflexia, imbalance, spasticity	Myelopathy, stroke
Mixed upper/lower motor neuron findings	Vitamin B_{12} deficiency
Trunk instability, wide base gait, ataxia	Cerebellar disease
Tremor, rigidity, bradykinesia	Parkinson's disease
Proximal weakness	Myopathies, PMR
Sensory deficits, acroparesthesias	Peripheral neuropathies
Cognitive impairment, poor judgment	Dementia (AD, others)
Focal motor/sensory deficits, cognitive decline	Vascular dementia, stroke
Memory loss, ataxia, urinary incontinence	Normal pressure hydrocephalus
History of falls with head trauma	SDH
Kyphosis	VCFs, camptocormia
Decreased ROM, joint deformities	Degenerative joint disease
Visual impairment	Glaucoma (peripheral), cataracts (blurred), macular degeneration (central)
Palpitations, chest pain, DOE	CHF, CAD, arrhythmias
Dizziness, vertigo	Vestibular problems, medication S/E
Drop attacks (sudden falls without dizziness/vertigo)	Vertebrobasilar insufficiency, seizures
Lightheadedness with sudden head turning	Carotid sinus hypersensitivity
Lightheadedness with sudden rise	Orthostatic hypotension (medication S/E)

Abbreviations: AD, Alzheimer disease; CAD, coronary artery disease; CHF, congestive heart failure; DOE, dyspnea on exertion; PMR, polymyalgia rheumatica; ROM, range of motion; S/E, side effects; SDH, subdural hematoma; VCF, vertebral compression fractures.

PREVENTION AND MANAGEMENT STRATEGIES
Nonpharmacologic

Exercise

The recommendations and general benefits of exercise in the older adult would generally include the incorporation of activities that maintain or increase flexibility, endurance, strength, and balance. In addition, an older adult with a medical condition for which exercise is therapeutic should perform exercises in a manner that treats the condition and should engage in physical activity in a manner that reduces the risk of developing other chronic diseases. Exercise plans should include a gradual (stepwise) approach to increase physical activity over time.[20] Muscle strengthening and weight-bearing activities are particularly important in the older adult given their role in preventing age-related loss of muscle mass, bone, and functional abilities.[20]

Meta-analyses have shown that exercising has consistent effects reducing falls in healthy older adult populations when prescribed and completed at the correct progression and intensity.[21,22] A 2009 Cochrane database review concluded that multiple-component group exercise programs reduced the rate of falls and risk of falling, as did Tai Chi and individually prescribed multiple-component home-based exercise programs.[11] A more recent meta-analysis concluded that exercise reduced the rate of falls in community-dwelling older people by 21%, with greater effects seen from exercise programs that challenged balance and involved more than 3 h/wk of duration. The investigators also found that exercise had a fall prevention effect in community-dwelling people with Parkinson's disease or cognitive impairment but no evidence of a fall prevention effect of exercise in residential care settings, among stroke survivors, or people recently discharged from the hospital.[21–23]

Masakazu and colleagues[24] compared the frequency of falls among 91 institutionalized frail elderly residents following three different interventions: (1) low-frequency exercise, (2) vitamin D supplementation, and (3) a combination of both. The intervention combining low-frequency exercise and vitamin D supplementation was the most effective for the reduction of falls among institutionalized frail elderly individuals.

From the public health and population management perspective, experts from Korea, Hong Kong, Taiwan, and Australia presented their research during the International Association of Gerontology and Geriatrics World Congress in Seoul (June 2013).[25] Meta-analyses presented revealed that in the elderly, Tai Chi is beneficial for balance improvement, and can lead to fall reductions (based on 13 randomized controlled trials). They recommended that communities should establish effective fall prevention programs; that exercise programs are an effective single prevention strategy; that environmental modifications are effective; and that multifactorial interventions, including exercise programs, can be recommended despite the need for more research.[25]

Specific exercise targets include strength, endurance, flexibility, and balance. A Cochrane review evaluating outcomes of these interventions revealed that programs targeting at least two of these components reduce the rate of falls. Furthermore, group exercises, such as Tai Chi and individually prescribed home exercise programs, are also effective. The role of physical therapy in targeting these strategies cannot be overstated.[11]

Environmental assessments and modifications

Environmental assessment and modification has proven to be effective preventing falls in community-dwelling older people. The training, experience, and approach of the individual performing the assessment and providing the recommendations are important factors in their effectiveness.[26]

Although nonspecific advice about modification of home hazards directed at untargeted groups of elderly persons has not been proven effective, standardized assessment of home hazards by an occupational therapist, along with specific recommendations and follow-up after hospital discharge, was associated with a 20% reduction in the risk of falling.[11,27] The most commonly recommended modifications in that study were the removal of rugs, a change to safer footwear, the use of nonslip bathmats, the use of lighting at night, and the addition of stair rails.[19] Evidence strongly supports the assessment and modification of the patient's home environment as part of a multifactorial fall prevention program, being particularly beneficial in high-risk individuals, such as those with prior history of falls.[11]

Pharmacologic

The concept of medication reconciliation and medication burden reduction has finally become standard of practice. Polypharmacy is commonplace in the elderly and it is not uncommon for patients to be treated by multiple medical providers with little to no coordination of care. Therefore, it is common to see medications prescribed to address side effects from other medications, resulting in a wide variety of problematic side effects and a large number of clinically important drug-drug interactions. Some common side effects include orthostatic hypotension, dizziness, and somnolence, all of which have been associated with falls. In one study, tapering and discontinuation of psychotropic medications, including benzodiazepines, other sleep medications, neuroleptic agents, and antidepressants, over a 14-week period was associated with a 39% reduction in the rate of falling.[28] Successful components of these interventions include review and possible reduction of medications.

SUMMARY

The clinical relevance of the multifactorial relationships of the deficits that lead to falls in older adults is that improvement in modifiable factors may help compensate for those functions or factors that are irreversibly affected.[3] Known effective strategies for reducing the number of older adult falls call for a multifactorial clinical approach, including gait and balance assessment, strength and balance exercises, environmental modifications, and medication review.[1] Implementing these on a large scale can prove to be challenging, as documented by investigators from the State Falls Prevention Project, a project funded by the Centers for Disease Control and Prevention, in which several state Departments of Health were charged with implementing clinical and community fall-prevention programs in specific geographic areas. Some of the challenges that they identified include difficulties and resistance to change physician practice, lack of program availability in many communities coupled with limited knowledge about their availability and value (when available), and long-term sustainability of these programs.[29]

Although there is no consensus about the optimal time to initiate screening, the rate of falling and the prevalence of risk factors for falling increase steeply after the age of 70 years.[2,30,31] Guidelines from several professional societies recommend that all elderly patients should be asked about any falls that have occurred during the previous year and should undergo clinical screenings of their gait and balance.[32] Health care providers play a crucial role in fall prevention by screening older adults for fall risk, reviewing and managing medications linked to falls, and recommending preventive strategies.

REFERENCES

1. Bergen G, Stevens MR, Burns ER. Falls and fall injuries among adults aged ≥ 65 years—United States, 2014. MMWR Morb Mortal Wkly Rep 2016;65(37):993–8.
2. Nevitt MC, Cummings SR, Hudes ES. Risk factors for injurious falls: a prospective study. J Gerontol 1991;46:M164–70.
3. Richardson JK. The confusing circular nature of falls research... and a possible antidote. Am J Phys Med Rehabil 2017;96:55–9.
4. Salzman B. Gait and balance disorders in older adults. Am Fam Physician 2010; 82(1):61–8.
5. Kearney FC, Harwood RH, Gladman JR, et al. The relationship between executive function and falls and gait abnormalities in older adults: a systematic review. Dement Geriatr Cogn Disord 2013;36:20–35.
6. Lord SR, Sherrington C, Menz HB, et al. Falls in older people: risk factors and strategies for prevention. Cambridge (United Kingdom): Cambridge University Press; 2007.
7. Shaw FE, Bond J, Richardson DA, et al. Multifactorial intervention after a fall in older people with cognitive impairment and dementia presenting to the accident and emergency department: randomised controlled trial. BMJ 2003; 326:73.

8. Booth V, Harwood R, Hood V, et al. Understanding the theoretical underpinning of the exercise component in a fall prevention programme for older adults with mild dementia: a realist review protocol. Syst Rev 2016;5:119.

9. NICE. Clinical Guideline 161. Falls: assessment and prevention of falls in older people. Available at: https://www.nice.org.uk/guidance/cg161. Accessed December 19, 2014.

10. Bloem BR, Haan J, Lagaay AM, et al. Investigation of gait in elderly subjects over 88 years of age. J Geriatr Psychiatry Neurol 1992;5(2):78–84.

11. Gillespie LD, Gillespie WJ, Robertson MC, et al. Interventions for preventing falls in elderly people. Cochrane Database Syst Rev 2009;(2):CD000340.

12. Zhang X-Y, Shuai J, Li L-P. Vision and relevant risk factor interventions for preventing falls among older people: a network meta-analysis. Sci Rep 2015;5:10559.

13. Grue EV, Kirkevold M, Mowinchel P, et al. Sensory impairment in hip fracture patients 65 years or older and effects of hearing/vision interventions on fall frequency. J Multidisc Healthcare 2008;2:1–11.

14. Leipzig RM, Cummin RG, Tineti ME. Drugs and falls in older people: a systematic review and meta-analysis: I. Psychotropic drugs. J Am Geriatr Soc 1999;47(1):30–9.

15. Leipzig RM, Cummin RG, Tineti ME. Drugs and falls in older people: a systematic review and meta-analysis: II. Cardiac and analgesic drugs. J Am Geriatr Soc 1999;47(1):40–50.

16. Delmonico MJ, Harris TB, Lee JS, et al. Alternative definitions of sarcopenia, lower extremity performance, and functional impairment with aging in older men and women. J Am Geriatr Soc 2007;55:769–74.

17. Doherty TJ. Aging and sarcopenia (invited review). J Appl Physiol 2003;95(4):1717–27.

18. Ganz DA, Bao Y, Shekelle PG, et al. Will my patient fall? JAMA 2007;297(1):77–86.

19. Tinetti ME. Preventing falls in elderly persons. N Engl J Med 2003;348:42–9.

20. Nelson ME, Rejeski WJ, Blair SN, et al. Physical activity and public health in older adults. recommendation from the American College of Sports Medicine and the American Heart Association. Circulation 2007;116:1094–105.

21. Sherrington C, Michaleff ZA, Fairhall N, et al. Exercise to prevent falls in older adults: an updated systematic review and meta-analysis. Br J Sports Med 2016. http://dx.doi.org/10.1136/bjsports-2016-096547.

22. Sherrington C, Tiedemann A, Fairhall N, et al. Exercise to prevent falls in older adults: an updated meta-analysis and best practice recommendations. N S W Public Health Bull 2011;22(4):78–83.

23. Sherrington C, Tiedemann A, Fairhall NJ, et al. Exercise for preventing falls in older people living in the community. Cochrane Database Syst Rev 2016;(11):CD012424.

24. Masakazu I, Higuchi Y, Todo E, et al. Low-frequency exercise and Vitamin D supplementation reduce falls among institutionalized frail elderly. Intl J Geront 2016;1–5.

25. Kim EJ, Arai H, Chan P, et al. Strategies on fall prevention for older people living in the community: a report from a round-table meeting in IAGG 2013. J Clin Geront Geriatr 2015;6:39–44.

26. Pighills A, Ballinger A, Pickering R, et al. A critical review of the effectiveness of environmental assessment and modification in the prevention of falls amongst community dwelling older people. Br J Occup Ther 2015;79(3):133–43.

27. Cummings RG, Thomas M, Szonyi G, et al. Home visits by an occupational therapist for assessment and modification of environmental hazards: a randomized trial of falls prevention. J Am Geriatr Soc 1999;47:1397–402.
28. Campbell AJ, Robertson MC, Gardner MM, et al. Psychotropic medication withdrawal and a homebased exercise program to prevent falls: a randomized, controlled trial. J Am Geriatr Soc 1999;47:850–3.
29. Shubert TE, Smith ML, Schneider EC, et al. Commentary: public health system perspective on implementation of evidence-based fall-prevention strategies for older adults. Front Public Health 2016;4:252.
30. Nevitt MC, Cummings SR, Kidd S, et al. Risk factors for recurrent non-syncopal falls: a prospective study. JAMA 1989;261:2663–8.
31. Sattin RW. Falls among older persons: a public health perspective. Annu Rev Public Health 1992;13:489–508.
32. American Geriatrics Society, British Geriatric Society, American Academy of Orthopaedic Surgeons Panel on Falls Prevention. Guideline for the prevention of falls in older persons. J Am Geriatr Soc 2001;49:664–72.

Geriatric Polypharmacy

Pharmacist as Key Facilitator in Assessing for Falls Risk: 2019 Update

Michelle A. Fritsch, PharmD[a],*, Penny S. Shelton, PharmD[b]

KEYWORDS

- Falls • Medication • Pharmacist • Geriatric • Falls assessment • Patient safety

KEY POINTS

- The health care burden associated with the growing incidence of falls among the elderly is anticipated to worsen.
- Pharmacists are members of the patient health care team not commonly thought of but uniquely positioned to help assess and address falls risk.
- Patients with positive falls screenings should be comprehensively assessed to identify and address multiple causative factors associated with falls.
- A 6-step, comprehensive falls assessment including falls-associated drugs and medical conditions is described, including implementation concepts based on pharmacy practice setting.

INTRODUCTION

Each year millions of falls-related injuries occur among individuals age 65 or older. As many as 1 in 3 older adults fall annually, and the toll from these falls generates a significant public health problem in the United States.[1] Falls often result in injuries, which require emergent care (2.5 million annually) and hospitalization (700,000 annually).[2] Falls-related injuries and subsequent debilitation can result in short- or long-term loss of independence.[3] Most tragically, despite much attention being focused on falls awareness, the falls death rate among older adults has continued to increase annually over the past decade, with an increase of approximately 7100 deaths between 2005 and 2011.[4] The Centers for Disease Control and Prevention (CDC) reported an adjusted direct medical cost for falls in 2013 as totaling $34 billion.[5,6] Because of the aging of our society, if significant proactive interventions are not put in place,

This is an update of an article that originally appeared in *Clinics in Geriatric Medicine*, Volume 33, Issue 2, May 2017.

[a] Meds MASH, LLC, 16326 Matthews Road, Monkton, MD 21111, USA; [b] North Carolina Association of Pharmacists, 1101 Slater Road, Suite 110, Durham, NC 27703, USA
* Corresponding author.
E-mail address: michelle@medsmash.com

both the number of and the costs to treat falls injuries are anticipated to continue to increase.

There are numerous factors proven to be associated with increased falls risk among the elderly. Medications are often implicated. Therefore, pharmacists can be instrumental in assessing and reducing falls risk. Falls and falls risk are particularly elevated during transitions of care, and pharmacists in both outpatient and inpatient settings have the ability to provide falls-risk reducing services.[7,8] Pharmacists' intensive education and training in medication therapy management are greatly needed to help improve patient safety.

In the outpatient setting, although commonplace for patients to see more than one physician or prescriber for their care, patients have been strongly encouraged to use one pharmacy. Using one pharmacy allows the pharmacist, after obtaining additional information regarding over-the-counter (OTC) medicines, herbal supplements, and illicit or recreational substances to review the entire medication regimen and identify actual or potential medication-related problems. This type of comprehensive medication therapy review can be conducted as part of an overall falls risk assessment and tailored to identify and address the use of falls risk-inducing drugs (FRIDs).

Pharmacists can do more than just identify falls risk. Casteel and colleagues[9] found pharmacists' recommendations for safer alternatives to reduce falls risk without compromising achievement of desired therapeutic goals. Another recent pilot program demonstrated the value of falls risk assessment within a community pharmacy setting, where identification of known FRIDs followed by medication change or dose-lowering recommendations resulted in a significant decrease in the use of FRIDs.[10] An analysis of falls prevention literature since 1994 found further evidence of the positive impact of pharmacist-conducted medication review.[11]

A well-conducted, pharmacist-provided falls assessment and intervention can make a difference; however, it is the opinion of the authors that in order to substantially improve the public health concerns associated with falls among the elderly, an interprofessional approach to the problem is required. Given that medications are frequently a culprit, pharmacists, regardless of practice setting, must proactively address falls risk as part of that interprofessional team, and the information gleaned from their falls-based assessment will frequently necessitate triage and patient referral for those who need further assessment and falls risk-reducing services (**Box 1**).

Box 1
The pharmacist as an interprofessional falls-risk reducing team member

The following are examples of frequent professionals to whom pharmacists may need to refer patients based on the falls assessment findings:
Physicians (eg, general practitioner, geriatrician, neurologist, endocrinologist, podiatrist)
　For appropriate workup of medical conditions as identified elsewhere in this publication
Physical therapist
　For strengthening and gait improvement
Occupational therapist
　For improvement in activities of daily living and in-home functioning and safety assessment
　For assessing patient for appropriate falls risk reduction aids
Home improvement handyman/contractor
　For assessment, building or renovating changes to reduce in-home falls hazards (assure contractor is licensed and insured and a certified aging-in-place specialist)

Falls happen in all settings and the morbidity and mortality, as well as direct and indirect costs associated with falls, have spurred the development of falls-related quality indicators in the care of patients. The Agency for Healthcare Research and Quality has called for improvement in the patient safety culture within hospitals, and the Center for Medicare and Medicaid's star ratings and quality measures on falls have elevated the importance of falls prevention among institutional settings, where inpatient and consultant pharmacists have become a vital resource for reducing falls and falls risk. The community pharmacist has long been acknowledged as the most accessible health care provider, which uniquely positions the pharmacist as the member of the health care team who can use their frequent interaction with patients to observe, assess, intervene, and monitor FRIDs as well as other falls risk factors. Today, most seniors live independently or with family members in the community; as previously noted, falling is highly prevalent among this population. However, less than half of patients who fall speak to their health care providers about falling[12]; therefore, it is critically important for pharmacists to proactively ask about and assess their patients for falls.

TOOLS FOR FALLS ASSESSMENT

There are several tools that have been developed and used to identify patients at risk for falls and to minimize those risks. A tool with objective measures, quantifiable scoring, and quick administration is preferred for an initial assessment. Many institutions and outpatient practices use tools to screen for falls risks. Patients identified to be at risk can then be assessed with a more in-depth tool to identify specific modifiable risk factors.

The Agency for Healthcare Research and Quality has made available an in-depth toolkit to assist hospitals with falls reduction. This multisystem toolkit is comprehensive and engages many practitioners within the hospital setting. It lacks specificity with FRIDs and risk-increasing medical conditions.[13] Similarly, the Johns Hopkins Falls Risk Assessment Tool is commonly used by nurses in the acute care setting due to ease of administration, but the tool lacks specificity for FRIDs and medical conditions.[14]

The CDC published the Stopping Elderly Accidents, Deaths, and Injuries (STEADI) Toolkit in 2015.[15] STEADI has been piloted within electronic medical record systems such as Epic and GE Centricity[16] and is proposed as a regular component of Medicare Annual Wellness Visits (MAWV) in the National Council on Aging Falls Free 2015 initiative.[17] In the STEADI toolkit, falls risk is addressed in an algorithmic fashion that designates the depth of assessment based on identified risks. The toolkit highlights the importance of certain commonly associated FRIDs without guidance for medication and medical condition screening and intervention. The sections addressing FRIDs and falls-associated medical conditions are limited to the most commonly associated with falls.

Furthermore, practitioners across the country use a variety of approaches to falls risk assessment. Both a lack of standardization and limited comprehensive elements within existing screening tools reduce the effectiveness of these screenings for individual patients.

In the fall of 2016, the American Society of Consultant Pharmacists and the National Council on Aging launched the Falls Risk Reduction Toolkit (http://www.ascp.com/fallstoolkit), intended to be a companion and enhancement to STEADI. This companion tool as introduced in the next section builds upon the screening elements of STEADI, allowing for a more comprehensive falls risk assessment and intervention.

PHARMACIST ASSESSMENT FOR FALLS

Taking a stepwise approach, a pharmacist can conduct a comprehensive falls risk assessment. Six key steps are proposed.

Step 1

There are some key initial indicators, which quickly orient a pharmacist or other provider to increased falls risk (**Fig. 1**). Age is an independent risk factor for falling.[18] Falls risk increases with advancing age. Falls increase at times immediately preceding, during, or following a care transition.[7,8] Transitions are prime times for confusion, greater debilitation, communication gaps, and medication errors, which can contribute to falls. Knowledge about a patient's living arrangements provides valuable insight regarding the patient's support network and availability or lack of important at-home safety resources. It is important for pharmacists to ask older adults about alcohol and other substances of abuse. Substance use disorders are a frequently unaddressed cause of falls among the older adult population.[19] Pharmacists can use the power of observation to identify mobility-related falls risk factors, such as the presence of an assistive ambulation device (eg, cane, walker, or arm of a caregiver), unsteady gait, or difficulty standing or rising from a chair. In addition, there are other common general signs associated with falling for which the pharmacist and other practitioners should assess (**Box 2, Table 1**).

Step 2

The number one predictor of a fall is a previous fall.[20] It is rare unless there is injury for patients to voluntarily share the occurrence of a fall. Often what health professionals

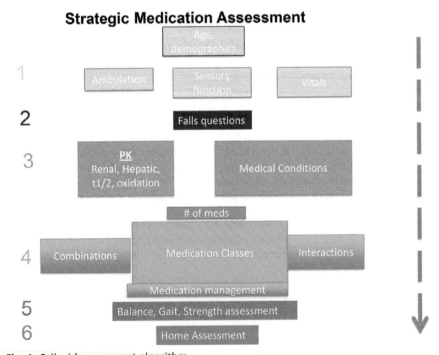

Fig. 1. Falls risk assessment algorithm.

> **Box 2**
> **Additional falls-related general signs or conditions**
>
> - Vital signs
>   - Blood pressure: assess for hypotension or orthostatic hypotension
>   - Heart rate: assess for any abnormal rate and rhythm
>   - Temperature: assess for fever (infection >>> confusion >>> fall)
>   - Pain: uncontrolled pain as distractor >>> falls
> - Sensory function
>   - Vision: use of assistive devices, last vision evaluation, impairments that cannot be corrected
>   - Hearing: use of assistive devices, last hearing evaluation if any evidence of impairment
>   - Taste/smell: impact on nutrition, strength, frailty
>   - Touch: neuropathy, especially of the lower extremities
> - Medication self-management—assess adherence, access, administration skills, and organization tool needs (mismanagement of medications >>> worsening of a falls-inducing medical condition and/or the occurrence of a falls-inducing adverse reaction)

would clearly define as a fall, patients will write-off as something other than a fall. "Oh, I didn't fall; I caught myself on the chair." For these reasons and others, it is important for pharmacists and other practitioners to ask about falls. Three key questions can be used to quickly screen for current falls risk and need for further assessment[15] (**Box 3**).

If a patient has experienced a fall, it is important to garner the patient's perspective as to the cause of the fall. At times, patients will be very uncertain as to the reason for their fall and claim "I don't know. All I know is the next minute I was on the floor." Other times patients may be able to speak to a specific cause: "my knee just gave out" or "I tripped over the living room rug" or "my chair tipped over when I was getting up." The more uncertainty as to the reason for the fall, the more likely there are to be causative factors completely unknown to the patient. This uncertainty will generally open up greater opportunities for assessment and patient education. However, just because the patient can point to a specific cause for their fall does not mean that the patient will not benefit from closer assessment and intervention. Falls are often multifactorial. A patient who seemingly fell due to tripping over clutter may have had their fall compounded by the presence of a balance-altering condition, FRID, or both.

Fear of falling alters how people live. Daily activities are limited or avoided; risk of isolation increases, and deconditioning can worsen.[21]

Step 3

There are several medical conditions that increase falls through physical function, neurologic, vascular, or pharmacokinetic changes. It is important for the pharmacist to educate patients regarding any falls-associated medical conditions as well as safety measures a patient can take to mitigate their risk (**Table 2**).

Step 4

Polypharmacy has been defined as 5 or more prescription medications.[75] Medication use in an aging population is a fine balance between evidence-based prescribing to sustain and enhance health and avoidance of inappropriate prescribing. Several tools have been designed and published to help guide appropriate prescribing. Some emphasize avoidance of medications with greater risk than efficacy.[76–79] Others emphasize inclusion of medications demonstrated to enhance health.[77] One such example is the evidence to support correction of vitamin D insufficiency.[11] With

Table 1
General assessment

General Patient Factors		
Age		
☐ Age over 65	☐ Age over 80	☐ Frail
Transition status		
☐ Pending transition	☐ Recent transition	
Living arrangements		
☐ Lives alone	☐ In-home care, full time	☐ In-home care, part time
☐ Lives with spouse or other	☐ Assisted living facility	☐ Skilled care facility
Substance use		
☐ Alcohol, ___ drinks per day	☐ Marijuana	☐ Other illicit substances
Vital signs		
Postural hypotension:	Pulse:	Pain:
☐ Systolic blood pressure (BP) falls ≥ −20 mm Hg	☐ Irregular	☐ Complaint of pain
☐ Diastolic BP falls ≥ −10 mm Hg	☐ <50 bpm	Pain location(s):
☐ Dizzy or lightheaded with standing	Temperature:	Pain score ___ (0–10)
	☐ Over 98.6°F	
Ambulation status		
☐ Cane	☐ Crutches	☐ Standard walker
☐ Front wheel walked	☐ Rollator	☐ Wheelchair
Sensory function		
Vision:	Hearing:	Feet/lower extremities:
☐ Acuity <20/40	☐ Hearing deficit	☐ Altered lower-extremity sensation
☐ Blurred vision	☐ Regular use hearing aid	☐ Foot pain
☐ No eye examination in last year	☐ Sporadic use hearing aid	☐ Bunion
☐ Corrected vision	Taste/smell:	☐ Hammer toe
☐ Regular use of glasses/contact lens	☐ Changes in taste	☐ Plantar fasciitis
☐ Sporadic use glasses/contacts	☐ Changes in smell	☐ Heel spur
		☐ Ingrown toenail
Medication self-management		
☐ Medications disorganized	☐ Evidence of adherence issues	

Box 3
Three quick screening questions for falls

1. Have you fallen in the past year?
    a. If yes, ask how many times and if there were any injuries.

2. Do you feel unsteady when standing or walking?

3. Do you worry about falling?

If the response is "yes" to any of these, then comprehensive assessment is warranted.

Data from Stevens JA, Phelan EA. Development of STEADI: a fall prevention resource for health care providers. Health Promot Pract 2013;14:710.

---

advancing age often comes an accumulation of medical conditions and health issues. Polypharmacy might be a reflection of overall health, or it may be a trigger to identify higher risk of inappropriate prescribing.[80]

In some instances, especially when FRIDs are involved, falls risk can increase even with fewer than 5 prescribed medications.[81,82] This risk further increases in patients with more advanced age, use of ambulation assistive devices, and overall poorer health.[83,84]

Changing medication regimens is a source of confusion, error, and adverse effects. A recent medication change can be a flag for pharmacist intervention.

The medication assessment starts with number of medications, determination of any recent medication changes, and an awareness of medication-related problems that can increase falls risk (**Table 3**).

The next step of the medication assessment is to look for medication classes that increase falls risk. Most of these have central nervous system (CNS) depressant, anticholinergic, hypoglycemic, or hypotensive effects (**Table 4**).

Step 5

For further falls risk assessment, there are 3 quick and relatively simple gait, strength, and balance assessments that provide objective evidence of falls risk (**Box 4**).

Step 6

The final step is to know what falls risk factors are present in the home. For those residing in assisted living or skilled nursing facilities, there is a team of providers assessing these risks. For those not living in an institutional setting, an environmental assessment allows identification and reduction of additional risks (**Box 5**).

OPERATIONALIZING PHARMACIST-CONDUCTED FALLS ASSESSMENT

The vision for the profession of pharmacy by 2020 calls for an advanced role for pharmacists in all patient care settings. Pharmacists, as members of the patient's health care team, will take on greater roles "in promoting wellness, preventing disease and contributing to disease management."[132] Falls risk assessment by pharmacists is one such advanced role. However, the infrastructure and payment models for advanced pharmacist-provided services have been challenging at best if not seemingly insurmountable barriers at times.

The assessment described above takes time. How does a pharmacist work this type of comprehensive service into their existing daily duties? Which patients does one target for screening or for a more comprehensive assessment? Depending on the

Table 2
Medical conditions associated with falls risk

Medical Conditions	Caveats
Arrhythmia (eg, atrial fibrillation, a fib)	Any rhythm abnormality increases falls risk; a fib has higher mortality[22–24]
Arthritis (osteo, rheumatoid)	Osteoarthritis of lower extremities highest risk; over time, strength & flexibility decline[25–27]; rheumatic conditions associated with fatigue and added falls risk during flare[28,29]
Cardiovascular disease	Rate or rhythm disturbance, impaired oxygenation and stamina all increase risk[30]; syncope; myocardial infarction with atypical heralding symptoms[31,32]
Cerebellar ataxia	Gait variability and falls risk[33]
Cerebrovascular accident (CVA)/Stroke	CVA and associated sequelae can impact balance, physical function, ambulation[34–36]
Dementia	Impact of Alzheimer disease and other dementias multifactorial, including brain atrophy, declining frontal cognitive functions, impact on sleep cycles, falls associated with multitasking difficulty[37,38]
Depression	Common comorbidity with chronic conditions; negatively impacts motivation, concentration, and planning[39–42]
Hemophilia	Brain or muscle bleeds, bleed in the joint can impair mobility[43]; fear of injury can lead to decreased physical stamina and fitness; hemophilia with incontinence has even higher falls risk[44]
Impaired hepatic function	Impact on dosing; monitor AST, ALT, CYP450 enzymes; alcohol has negative impact on hepatic function and falls risk[45]; nonalcoholic fatty liver disease,[46] cirrhosis, hepatic encephalopathy with elevated ammonia levels associated with falls[47,48]
Impaired renal function	Renal impairment impacts clearance of medications, therapeutic and adverse effects; hemodialysis associated with falls risk[49,50]
Incontinence	Rush to bathroom, nocturia (with other risks of ambulating at night quickly in the dark with rapid standing not fully awake), urgency, urinary tract infections (UTIs) increase falls risk[51–53]
Infection (eg, UTI)	Confusion common symptom of infection; infections with most evidence of falls risk are UTI, bronchitic, pneumonia[54,55]
Lower extremity issue	Arthroplasty (especially first 1–3 d postoperative), neuropathy, injury, pain, physical changes, wounds, weakness all associated with falls (others); assure ambulation assistive device used correctly[56–63]
Malnutrition	Risk factors of muscle mass loss, weakness, associated cognitive decline, reduced concentration, sedation, reduced energy and stamina[64,65]
Multiple sclerosis	Annual fall rate near 60%; multifactorial[66,67]
Obesity	Associated with sedentary lifestyle, decreased strength, flexibility, stamina, muscle atrophy; may be associated with lower socioeconomic status, chronic health conditions, pain, anxiety, depression[68,69]
Parkinson disease	Orthostatic hypotension, gradually increasing imbalance, freezing, on/off phenomenon, impaired cognition[70,71]
Seizures	Syncopal and ictal episodes, especially if associated with loss of consciousness[72,73]; ictal bradyarrhythmias as a form of arrhythmogenic epilepsy[74]

Table 3
General medication assessment

Medication Review		
Number of medications (Rx, as needed, OTC, vitamin, supplement, herbal)	☐ ≥5	☐ ≥10
Recent medication regimen change	☐ Within last week	☐ Within last month
Falls risk medication-related problems detected:		
☐ Suboptimal dose[a] ☐ Interactions between medications, food, medical conditions ☐ Allergies and intolerances within current regimen	☐ Dose too high[b] ☐ Lacking medication therapy for all medication-requiring indications ☐ Unnecessary medication	☐ Safer evidence-based therapy available ☐ Difficulty administering medication[c]

[a] Suboptimal dose - check doses based on renal and hepatic function.
[b] Dose too high - causing adverse effects and/or unnecessary risk.
[c] Eye drops, inhalers, large dosage forms.

setting in which the pharmacist works, it may be wise to partner with others in carrying out various components of the assessment.

In the hospital, depending on patient data and falls metrics for the facility, it may be prudent to include a pharmacist in the assessment of any patient who is seen in the emergency department beause of a fall-related injury. The number one predictor of falling is a recent history of a fall.[20] Therefore, in the emergency department, if the causative factors are not initially and adequately addressed, another fall and subsequent emergency room visit or hospitalization is likely to occur. Inpatient pharmacists at the time of dispensing can flag FRIDs before initial administration, such that appropriate precautions can be put in place on the floor to prevent an in-hospital fall. When appropriate, safer alternatives can be recommended by the inpatient pharmacist. Before discharge, pharmacists can help provide patient education on appropriate use of medications and safety precautions to help minimize falls risk after hospitalization. In addition, pharmacists are important individuals to include on patient education committees, which may be responsible for designing or selecting falls risk education materials for patients and caregivers.

The long-term-care operational pharmacist can screen initial orders, on a skilled or assisted-living new patient admission, for FRIDs and alert the nursing and medical staff to not only the risk, but also potentially safer options. The consultant pharmacist in these postacute and long-term-care settings can review patient-specific falls-related information from the Minimum Data Set (MDS) 3.0,[133] as well as patient care notes, and participate in care planning to design a team-based approach to falls risk reduction.

In the outpatient setting, pharmacists who are embedded in ambulatory care practices have frequently been found to improve patient outcomes for diabetes, hypertension, hyperlipidemia, and anticoagulation services. More recently, pharmacists in collaboration with medical practices have become more involved in screening and preventative services, such as the MAWV.[134] A brief falls screening is part of the MAWV. Pharmacists can be instrumental in helping a medical practice conduct more comprehensive follow-up to problems detected during the wellness check. Pharmacists are especially beneficial for problems such as falls that are commonly known to be associated with medications.

Table 4
Medication review

Medication Class	Type	Effects
Anticholinergic	Anticholinergic (eg, oxybutynin, trihexiphenidyl, amitryptyline, antihistamines)	Dry eyes impact vision, dry mouth increases beverage consumption leading to frequent urination, CNS depression, constipation[85–87]
CNS depressant	Benzodiazepines (short or long t$_{1/2}$)	Consistent evidence of increased falls risk with all benzodiazepines; slow carefully monitored taper required for withdrawal of therapy[88–91]
	Antidepressants	Tricyclic agents have anticholinergic effects; selective serotonin reuptake inhibitors associated with fragility fractures and with falls; citalopram increases QTc interval; most require slow taper to withdraw[92–95]
	Sedative/hypnotics	Sleep cycles change with aging; typical requirement 7–8 h; agents impair gait, balance, equilibrium, can have amnestic effect, impaired motor vehicle operation[89,96]; consider melatonin 1–2 mg 1 h before bedtime[97]
	Antipsychotics/neuroleptics—typical or atypical	Typical agents primary mechanism with dopamine-associated with motor & extrapyramidal symptoms; atypical agents also associated with falls with mechanism more involving serotonin; risk similar among available atypical agents[98–100]
	Anticonvulsant	Associated with decreased bone density[101,102]; use associated with falls and fractures[103]; risk of seizure increases with medication or dosing changes[104,105]
	Muscle relaxant	Not well-tolerated and limited evidence of efficacy; highly associated with falls[106,107]
	Opioids	CNS depressant effects, [108–112] constipation, taper slowly to withdraw with use over a few days[113]
	OTC: diphenhydramine, doxylamine	Sedating antihistamines and OTC sedatives are highly anticholinergic with CNS depressant effects[114]; use nonsedating antihistamines for allergies
Cardiovascular/endocrine	Antihypertensive/cardiovascular (CV) medications	Orthostatic hypotension, postural dizziness—assess orthostatic BP[115,116], include diet, weight management, [117] sleep apnea treatment in overall plan; goal is to treat to current guidelines to minimize CV risk while avoiding hypotension[118,119]
	Hypoglycemia agents	Insulin and sulfonylureas most associated with hypoglycemia; long-term metformin associated with B12 deficiency neuropathy[120–124]

Data from https://www.cms.gov/Medicare/Prescription-Drug-Coverage/PrescriptionDrugCovGenIn/Downloads/2016-Star-Ratings-User-Call-Slides-v2015_08_05.pdf. Accessed February 8, 2017.

> **Box 4**
> **Gait, balance, strength**
>
> Timed Up and Go test $\geq$12 seconds[125–127]
>
> 30-second chair stand test below average score (scoring table with tool in STEADI)[128,129]
>
> 4-Stage balance test full tandem stance less than 10 seconds[130,131]
>
> Observed gait problems or difficulty standing

Community pharmacists could establish an FRIDs component to their existing medication therapy management services or develop a separate service that could help build business for the pharmacy while improving the care of their patients. Because falling and falls injuries are frequently a cause of loss of independence, a community-based falls-assessment service has the potential to help patients age in

> **Box 5**
> **Environmental assessment**
>
> *Bathroom:*
>
> - Shower: lip or ledge to climb in
>   - Surface, nonslip
>   - Grab bars
> - Toilet: raise seat if needed
>   - Grab bars
> - Space: wheelchair or walker accessible if needed
>
> *Bedroom:*
>
> - Bed: height, bed rail if needed
> - Eyeglasses within reach
> - Night light
> - Accessibility to bathroom or bedside commode
>
> *Kitchen*
>
> - Ability to reach cabinets, pantry
> - Safety of step stool if needed
>
> *Steps/stairs*
>
> - Height
> - Sturdy rails
> - Surface: nonslip or trip
> - Adequate lighting
>
> *All rooms*
>
> - Open flow to ambulate between rooms and key spaces
>   - Clutter and furniture out of path
> - Electrical cords out of walking path
> - Blind cords out of walking path
> - Surfaces nonslip or trip
> - Rugs removed or secured to floor

place more safely. Community pharmacists may want to set patient appointments for this type of service. Before an appointment, a technician could print out available and pertinent patient information for the pharmacist to review before or during the appointment. Community pharmacists could partner with aging services in the community as well as local care managers who could conduct initial falls screenings and refer appropriate patients to the pharmacist for a more comprehensive assessment. A community pharmacy may choose to train technicians or clerks to ask falls screening questions when interacting with patients at the time of medication pickup or delivery. Positive screenings could be reported back to the pharmacist for further action. Pharmacies could use electronic tablets preloaded with a falls screening question application. Patients or caregivers could self-screen and self-report to ask for further assessment.

SUMMARY

Falls frequently occur among the aging population, resulting in significant and sometimes fatal health consequences. Because of the aging of society, both the incidence and the cost of falls are anticipated to increase. Multiple factors, including medications, are commonly associated with falls in this patient population. Wherever older adults receive care, pharmacists are members of the patient health care team uniquely positioned to help assess and address falls risk. Comprehensive assessment such as the step-wise approach described within this article is needed to adequately identify and address multiple factors associated with falls in this population.

REFERENCES

1. Tromp AM, Pluijm SM, Smit JH, et al. Fall-risk screening test: a prospective study on predictors for falls in community-dwelling elderly. J Clin Epidemiol 2001; 54(8):837–44.
2. Centers for Disease Control and Prevention. Important facts about falls. Available at: http://www.cdc.gov/homeandrecreationalsafety/falls/adultfalls.html. Accessed June 19, 2016.
3. Tinetti ME, Williams CS. Falls, injuries due to falls, and the risk of admission to a nursing home. N Engl J Med 1997;337(18):1279–84.
4. Morbidity and Mortality Weekly Report. CDC National Health Report: leading causes of morbidity and mortality and associated behavioral risk and protective factors—United States, 2005–2013. Available at: http://www.cdc.gov/mmwr/preview/mmwrhtml/su6304a2.htm. Accessed June 20, 2016.
5. Centers for Disease Control and Prevention. Cost of falls among older adults. Available at: http://www.cdc.gov/homeandrecreationalsafety/falls/fallcost.html. Accessed June 19, 2016.
6. Stevens JA, Corso PS, Finkelstein EA, et al. The costs of fatal and nonfatal falls among older adults. Inj Prev 2006;12:290–5.
7. Stitt DM, Elliott DP, Thompson SN. Medication discrepancies identified at time of hospital discharge in a geriatric population. Am J Geriatr Pharmacother 2011; 9(4):234–40.
8. Mixon AS, Myers AP, Leak CL, et al. Characteristics associated with postdischarge medication errors. Mayo Clin Proc 2014;89(8):1042–51.
9. Casteel C, Blalock SJ, Ferreri S, et al. Implementation of a community pharmacy-based falls prevention program. Am J Geriatr Pharmacother 2011; 9(5):310–9.e2.

10. Mott DA, Martin B, Breslow R, et al. Impact of a medication therapy management intervention targeting medications associated with falling: results of a pilot study. J Am Pharm Assoc (2003) 2016;56(1):22–8.

11. Stevens JA, Lee R. The Potential to Reduce Falls and Avert Costs by Clinically Managing Fall Risk. Am J Prev Med 2018;55(3):290–7.

12. Stevens JA, Ballesteros MF, Mack KA, et al. Gender differences in seeking care for falls in the aged medicare population. Am J Prev Med 2012;43:59–62.

13. RAND Corporation, Boston University School of Public Health, ECRI Institute. Agency for Healthcare Research and Quality. Preventing falls in hospitals: a toolkit for improving quality of care. Available at: http://www.ahrq.gov/professionals/systems/hospital/fallpxtoolkit/index.html. Accessed June 20, 2016.

14. Johns Hopkins falls risk assessment tool. Available at: http://www.hopkinsmedicine.org/institute_nursing/models_tools/Appendix%20A_JHFRAT.pdf. Accessed June 20, 2016.

15. Stevens JA, Phelan EA. Development of STEADI: a fall prevention resource for health care providers. Health Promot Pract 2013;14:706–14.

16. National Falls Prevention Resource Center. Center for Healthy Aging. National Council on Aging. STEADI implementation and partnering with health care. Available at: https://www.ncoa.org/wp-content/uploads/STEADI-Webinar-Slidedeck.pdf. Accessed June 20, 2016.

17. National Council on Aging. The 2015 Falls Free National Action Plan. Available at: https://www.ncoa.org/resources/2015-falls-free-national-falls-prevention-action-plan/. Accessed June 20, 2016.

18. Gillespie LD, Robertson MC, Gillespie WJ, et al. Interventions for preventing falls in older people living in the community. Cochrane Database Syst Rev 2012;(9):CD007146.

19. National Council on Alcoholism and Drug Dependence, Inc. An Invisible Epidemic: alcoholism and drug dependence among older adults. Available at: http://www.ncadd.org/images/stories/PDF/factsheet-alcoholismanddrug dependenceamongolderadults.pdf. Accessed June 20, 2016.

20. American Geriatrics Society. Prevention of falls in older persons: AGS/BGS clinical practice guidelines 2010. Available at: http://www.medcats.com/FALLS/frameset.htm. Accessed June 20, 2016.

21. Lachman ME, Howland J, Tennstedt S, et al. Fear of falling and activity restriction: the survey of activities and fear of falling in the elderly (SAFE). J Gerontol B Psychol Sci Soc Sci 1998;53:P43Y50.

22. O'Neal WT, Qureshi WT, Judd SE, et al. Effect of falls on frequency of atrial fibrillation and mortality risk (from the REasons for Geographic And Racial Differences in Stroke Study). Am J Cardiol 2015;116(8):1213–8.

23. Jansen S, Kenny RA, de Rooij SE, et al. Self-reported cardiovascular conditions are associated with falls and syncope in community-dwelling older adults. Age Ageing 2015;44(3):525–9.

24. Jansen S, Frewen J, Finucane C, et al. AF is associated with self-reported syncope and falls in a general population cohort. Age Ageing 2015;44(4):598–603.

25. Ng CT, Tan MP. Osteoarthritis and falls in the older person. Age Ageing 2013; 42(5):561–6.

26. Doré AL, Golightly YM, Mercer VS, et al. Lower-extremity osteoarthritis and the risk of falls in a community-based longitudinal study of adults with and without osteoarthritis. Arthritis Care Res (Hoboken) 2015;67(5):633–9.

27. Scott D, Blizzard L, Fell J, et al. Prospective study of self-reported pain, radiographic osteoarthritis, sarcopenia progression, and falls risk in community-dwelling older adults. Arthritis Care Res (Hoboken) 2012;64(1):30–7.

28. Brenton-Rule A, Dalbeth N, Bassett S, et al. The incidence and risk factors for falls in adults with rheumatoid arthritis: a systematic review. Semin Arthritis Rheum 2015;44(4):389–98.

29. Stanmore EK, Oldham J, Skelton DA, et al. Risk factors for falls in adults with rheumatoid arthritis: a prospective study. Arthritis Care Res (Hoboken) 2013; 65(8):1251–8.

30. Gnjidic D, Bennett A, Le Couteur DG, et al. Ischemic heart disease, prescription of optimal medical therapy and geriatric syndromes in community-dwelling older men: a population-based study. Int J Cardiol 2015;192:49–55.

31. Grosmaitre P, Le Vavasseur O, Yachouh E, et al. Significance of atypical symptoms for the diagnosis and management of myocardial infarction in elderly patients admitted to emergency departments. Arch Cardiovasc Dis 2013;106(11): 586–92.

32. Frisoli A Jr, Ingham SJ, Paes ÂT, et al. Frailty predictors and outcomes among older patients with cardiovascular disease: data from Fragicor. Arch Gerontol Geriatr 2015;61(1):1–7.

33. Schniepp R, Wuehr M, Schlick C, et al. Increased gait variability is associated with the history of falls in patients with cerebellar ataxia. J Neurol 2014;261(1): 213–23.

34. Jalayondeja C, Sullivan PE, Pichaiyongwongdee S. Six-month prospective study of fall risk factors identification in patients post-stroke. Geriatr Gerontol Int 2014; 14(4):778–85.

35. Tsang CS, Liao LR, Chung RC, et al. Psychometric properties of the Mini-Balance Evaluation Systems Test (Mini-BESTest) in community-dwelling individuals with chronic stroke. Phys Ther 2013;93(8):1102–15.

36. Minet LR, Peterson E, von Koch L, et al. Occurrence and predictors of falls in people with stroke: six-year prospective study. Stroke 2015;46(9):2688–90.

37. Mignardot JB, Beauchet O, Annweiler C, et al. Postural sway, falls, and cognitive status: a cross-sectional study among older adults. J Alzheimers Dis 2014; 41(2):431–9.

38. Epstein NU, Guo R, Farlow MR, et al. Medication for Alzheimer's disease and associated fall hazard: a retrospective cohort study from the Alzheimer's disease neuroimaging initiative. Drugs Aging 2014;31(2):125–9.

39. Stuart AL, Pasco JA, Jacka FN, et al. Falls and depression in men: a population-based study. Am J Mens Health 2015. [Epub ahead of print].

40. Kvelde T, Lord SR, Close JC, et al. Depressive symptoms increase fall risk in older people, independent of antidepressant use, and reduced executive and physical functioning. Arch Gerontol Geriatr 2015;60(1):190–5.

41. Launay C, De Decker L, Annweiler C, et al. Association of depressive symptoms with recurrent falls: a cross-sectional elderly population based study and a systematic review. J Nutr Health Aging 2013;17(2):152–7.

42. Lohman MC, Mezuk B, Dumenci L. Depression and frailty: concurrent risks for adverse health outcomes. Aging Ment Health 2015;1–10.

43. Fearn M, Hill K, Williams S, et al. Balance dysfunction in adults with haemophilia. Haemophilia 2010;16(4):606–14.

44. Sammels M, Vandesande J, Vlaeyen E, et al. Falling and fall risk factors in adults with haemophilia: an exploratory study. Haemophilia 2014;20(6):836–45.

45. Wadd S, Papadopoulos C. Drinking behaviour and alcohol-related harm amongst older adults: analysis of existing UK datasets. BMC Res Notes 2014; 7:741.

46. Bertolotti M, Lonardo A, Mussi C, et al. Nonalcoholic fatty liver disease and aging: epidemiology to management. World J Gastroenterol 2014;20(39): 14185–204.

47. Román E, Córdoba J, Torrens M, et al. Falls and cognitive dysfunction impair health-related quality of life in patients with cirrhosis. Eur J Gastroenterol Hepatol 2013;25(1):77–84.

48. Soriano G, Román E, Córdoba J, et al. Cognitive dysfunction in cirrhosis is associated with falls: a prospective study. Hepatology 2012;55(6):1922–30.

49. McAdams-DeMarco MA, Suresh S, Law A, et al. Frailty and falls among adult patients undergoing chronic hemodialysis: a prospective cohort study. BMC Nephrol 2013;14:224.

50. López-Soto PJ, De Giorgi A, Senno E, et al. Renal disease and accidental falls: a review of published evidence. BMC Nephrol 2015;16(1):176.

51. Luo X, Chuang CC, Yang E, et al. Prevalence, management and outcomes of medically complex vulnerable elderly patients with urinary incontinence in the United States. Int J Clin Pract 2015;69(12):1517–24.

52. Bresee C, Dubina ED, Khan AA, et al. Prevalence and correlates of urinary incontinence among older community-dwelling women. Female Pelvic Med Reconstr Surg 2014;20(6):328–33.

53. Godmaire GC, Grenier S, Tannenbaum C. An independent association between urinary incontinence and falls in chronic benzodiazepine users. J Am Geriatr Soc 2015;63(5):1035–7.

54. Infectious Diseases Society of America. Tripped up by a bug: infection may cause falls, especially in older people, study suggests. ScienceDaily 2015. Available at: www.sciencedaily.com/releases/2015/10/151009155255.htm. Accessed June 20, 2016.

55. Limpawattana P, Phungoen P, Mitsungnern T, et al. Atypical presentations of older adults at the emergency department and associated factors. Arch Gerontol Geriatr 2016;62:97–102.

56. Zak M, Krupnik S, Puzio G, et al. Assessment of functional capability and ongoing falls-risk in older institutionalized people after total hip arthroplasty for femoral neck fractures. Arch Gerontol Geriatr 2015;61(1):14–20.

57. Mallinson T, Leland NE, Chan TH. The need for uniform quality reporting across post-acute care rehabilitation settings: an examination of accidental falls. J Am Geriatr Soc 2015;63(1):195–7.

58. Matsumoto H, Okuno M, Nakamura T, et al. Incidence and risk factors for falling in patients after total knee arthroplasty compared to healthy elderly individuals. Yonago Acta Med 2014;57(4):137–45.

59. Swinkels A, Newman JH, Allain TJ. A prospective observational study of falling before and after knee replacement surgery. Age Ageing 2009;38(2):175–81.

60. Gell NM, Wallace RB, LaCroix AZ, et al. Mobility device use in older adults and incidence of falls and worry about falling: findings from the 2011-2012 national health and aging trends study. J Am Geriatr Soc 2015;63(5):853–9.

61. Toosizadeh N, Mohler J, Armstrong DG, et al. The influence of diabetic peripheral neuropathy on local postural muscle and central sensory feedback balance control. PLoS One 2015;10(8):e0135255.

62. Callaghan B, Kerber K, Langa KM, et al. Longitudinal patient-oriented outcomes in neuropathy: importance of early detection and falls. Neurology 2015;85(1): 71–9.

63. Johnson RL, Duncan CM, Ahn KS, et al. Fall-prevention strategies and patient characteristics that impact fall rates after total knee arthroplasty. Anesth Analg 2014;119(5):1113–8.

64. Westergren A, Hagell P, Sjödahl Hammarlund C. Malnutrition and risk of falling among elderly without home-help service–a cross sectional study. J Nutr Health Aging 2014;18(10):905–11.

65. Meijers JM, Halfens RJ, Neyens JC, et al. Predicting falls in elderly receiving home care: the role of malnutrition and impaired mobility. J Nutr Health Aging 2012;16(7):654–8.

66. Hoang PD, Cameron MH, Gandevia SC, et al. Neuropsychological, balance, and mobility risk factors for falls in people with multiple sclerosis: a prospective cohort study. Arch Phys Med Rehabil 2014;95(3):480–6.

67. Coote S, Finlayson M, Sosnoff JJ. Level of mobility limitations and falls status in persons with multiple sclerosis. Arch Phys Med Rehabil 2014;95(5):862–6.

68. Mitchell RJ, Lord SR, Harvey LA, et al. Obesity and falls in older people: mediating effects of disease, sedentary behavior, mood, pain and medication use. Arch Gerontol Geriatr 2015;60(1):52–8.

69. Mitchell RJ, Lord SR, Harvey LA, et al. Associations between obesity and overweight and fall risk, health status and quality of life in older people. Aust N Z J Public Health 2014;38(1):13–8.

70. Paul SS, Allen NE, Sherrington C, et al. Risk factors for frequent falls in people with Parkinson's disease. J Parkinsons Dis 2014;4(4):699–703.

71. Paul SS, Canning CG, Sherrington C, et al. Three simple clinical tests to accurately predict falls in people with Parkinson's disease. Mov Disord 2013;28(5): 655–62.

72. Nguyen-Michel VH, Bornand A, Balathazar AM, et al. Fall related to epileptic seizures in the elderly. Epileptic Disord 2015;17(3):287–91.

73. Homann B, Plaschg A, Grundner M, et al. The impact of neurological disorders on the risk for falls in the community dwelling elderly: a case-controlled study. BMJ Open 2013;3(11):e003367.

74. Kepez A, Erdogan O. Arrhythmogenic epilepsy and pacing need: a matter of controversy. World J Clin Cases 2015;3(10):872–5.

75. Gnjidic D, Hilmer SN, Blyth FM, et al. Polypharmacy cutoff and outcomes: five or more medicines were used to identify community-dwelling older men at risk of different adverse outcomes. J Clin Epidemiol 2012;65(9):989–95.

76. By the American Geriatrics Society 2015 Beers Criteria Update Expert Panel. American Geriatrics Society 2015 Updated Beers Criteria for potentially inappropriate medication use in older adults. J Am Geriatr Soc 2015;63(11):2227–46.

77. Gallagher P, Ryan C, Byrne S, et al. STOPP (Screening Tool of Older Person's Prescriptions) and START (Screening Tool to Alert doctors to Right Treatment). Consensus validation. Int J Clin Pharmacol Ther 2008;46(2):72–83.

78. Hill-Taylor B, Sketris I, Hayden J, et al. Application of the STOPP/START criteria: a systematic review of the prevalence of potentially inappropriate prescribing in older adults, and evidence of clinical, humanistic and economic impact. J Clin Pharm Ther 2013;38(5):360–72.

79. Fitzgerald LS, Hanlon JT, Shelton PS, et al. Reliability of a modified medication appropriateness index in ambulatory older persons. Ann Pharmacother 1997; 31(5):543–8.

80. Fried TR, O'Leary J, Towle V, et al. Health outcomes associated with polypharmacy in community-dwelling older adults: a systematic review. J Am Geriatr Soc 2014;62(12):2261–72.
81. Laflamme L, Monárrez-Espino J, Johnell K, et al. Type, number or both? A population-based matched case-control study on the risk of fall injuries among older people and number of medications beyond fall-inducing drugs. PLoS One 2015;10(3):e0123390.
82. Helgadóttir B, Laflamme L, Monárrez-Espino J, et al. Medication and fall injury in the elderly population; do individual demographics, health status and lifestyle matter? BMC Geriatr 2014;14:92.
83. Ham AC, Swart KM, Enneman AW, et al. Medication-related fall incidents in an older, ambulant population: the B-PROOF study. Drugs Aging 2014;31(12):917–27.
84. Thorell K, Ranstad K, Midlöv P, et al. Is use of fall risk-increasing drugs in an elderly population associated with an increased risk of hip fracture, after adjustment for multimorbidity level: a cohort study. BMC Geriatr 2014;14:131.
85. Richardson K, Bennett K, Maidment ID, et al. Use of medications with anticholinergic activity and self-reported injurious falls in older community-dwelling adults. J Am Geriatr Soc 2015;63(8):1561–9.
86. Landi F, Dell'Aquila G, Collamati A, et al. Anticholinergic drug use and negative outcomes among the frail elderly population living in a nursing home. J Am Med Dir Assoc 2014;15(11):825–9.
87. Crispo JA, Willis AW, Thibault DP, et al. Associations between anticholinergic burden and adverse health outcomes in Parkinson disease. PLoS One 2016;11(3):e0150621.
88. de Vries OJ, Peeters G, Elders P, et al. The elimination half-life of benzodiazepines and fall risk: two prospective observational studies. Age Ageing 2013;42(6):764–70.
89. Allain H, Bentué-Ferrer D, Polard E, et al. Postural instability and consequent falls and hip fractures associated with use of hypnotics in the elderly: a comparative review. Drugs Aging 2005;22(9):749–65.
90. Guaiana G, Barbui C. Discontinuing benzodiazepines: best practices. Epidemiol Psychiatr Sci 2016;25(3):214–6.
91. Darker CD, Sweeney BP, Barry JM, et al. Psychosocial interventions for benzodiazepine harmful use, abuse or dependence. Cochrane Database Syst Rev 2015;(5):CD009652.
92. Sultana J, Spina E, Trifirò G. Antidepressant use in the elderly: the role of pharmacodynamics and pharmacokinetics in drug safety. Expert Opin Drug Metab Toxicol 2015;11(6):883–92.
93. Boyce RD, Handler SM, Karp JF, et al. Age-related changes in antidepressant pharmacokinetics and potential drug-drug interactions: a comparison of evidence-based literature and package insert information. Am J Geriatr Pharmacother 2012;10(2):139–50.
94. Coupland CA, Dhiman P, Barton G, et al. A study of the safety and harms of antidepressant drugs for older people: a cohort study using a large primary care database. Health Technol Assess 2011;15(28):1–202, iii–iv.
95. Kerse N, Flicker L, Pfaff JJ, et al. Falls, depression and antidepressants in later life: a large primary care appraisal. PLoS One 2008;3(6):e2423.
96. Gunja N. In the Zzz zone: the effects of Z-drugs on human performance and driving. J Med Toxicol 2013;9(2):163–71.

97. Vural EM, van Munster BC, de Rooij SE. Optimal dosages for melatonin supplementation therapy in older adults: a systematic review of current literature. Drugs Aging 2014;31(6):441–51.

98. Chatterjee S, Chen H, Johnson ML, et al. Risk of falls and fractures in older adults using atypical antipsychotic agents: a propensity score-adjusted, retrospective cohort study. Am J Geriatr Pharmacother 2012;10(2):83–94.

99. Mehta S, Chen H, Johnson ML, et al. Risk of falls and fractures in older adults using antipsychotic agents: a propensity-matched retrospective cohort study. Drugs Aging 2010;27(10):815–29.

100. Lavsa SM, Fabian TJ, Saul MI, et al. Influence of medications and diagnoses on fall risk in psychiatric inpatients. Am J Health Syst Pharm 2010;67(15):1274–80.

101. Gold PW, Pavlatou MG, Michelson D, et al. Chronic administration of anticonvulsants but not antidepressants impairs bone strength: clinical implications. Transl Psychiatry 2015;5:e576.

102. Carbone LD, Johnson KC, Robbins J, et al. Antiepileptic drug use, falls, fractures, and BMD in postmenopausal women: findings from the women's health initiative (WHI). J Bone Miner Res 2010;25(4):873–81.

103. Shiek Ahmad B, Hill KD, O'Brien TJ, et al. Falls and fractures in patients chronically treated with antiepileptic drugs. Neurology 2012;79(2):145–51.

104. Saengsuwan J, Laohasiriwong W, Boonyaleepan S, et al, Integrated Epilepsy Research Group. Seizure-related vehicular crashes and falls with injuries for people with epilepsy (PWE) in northeastern Thailand. Epilepsy Behav 2014; 32:49–54.

105. Classen S, Crizzle AM, Winter SM, et al. Evidence-based review on epilepsy and driving. Epilepsy Behav 2012;23(2):103–12.

106. Spence MM, Shin PJ, Lee EA, et al. Risk of injury associated with skeletal muscle relaxant use in older adults. Ann Pharmacother 2013;47(7–8):993–8.

107. IBillups SJ, Delate T, Hoover B. Injury in an elderly population before and after initiating a skeletal muscle relaxant. Ann Pharmacother 2011;45(4):485–91.

108. Pergolizzi J, Böger RH, Budd K, et al. Opioids and the management of chronic severe pain in the elderly: consensus statement of an International Expert Panel with focus on the six clinically most often used World Health Organization Step III opioids (buprenorphine, fentanyl, hydromorphone, methadone, morphine, oxycodone). Pain Pract 2008;8(4):287–313.

109. Söderberg KC, Laflamme L, Möller J. Newly initiated opioid treatment and the risk of fall-related injuries. A nationwide, register-based, case-crossover study in Sweden. CNS Drugs 2013;27(2):155–61.

110. O'Neil CK, Hanlon JT, Marcum ZA. Adverse effects of analgesics commonly used by older adults with osteoarthritis: focus on non-opioid and opioid analgesics. Am J Geriatr Pharmacother 2012;10(6):331–42.

111. Rolita L, Spegman A, Tang X, et al. Greater number of narcotic analgesic prescriptions for osteoarthritis is associated with falls and fractures in elderly adults. J Am Geriatr Soc 2013;61(3):335–40.

112. Dowell D, Haegerich TM, Chou R. CDC guideline for prescribing opioids for chronic pain—United States, 2016. MMWR Recomm Rep 2016;65:1–49.

113. Hao J, Lucido D, Cruciani RA. Potential impact of abrupt opioid therapy discontinuation in the management of chronic pain: a pilot study on patient perspective. J Opioid Manag 2014;10(1):9–20.

114. Albert SM, Roth T, Toscani M, et al. Sleep health and appropriate use of OTC sleep aids in older adults—recommendations of a Gerontological Society of America Workgroup. Gerontologist 2015. [Epub ahead of print].

115. Zia A, Kamaruzzaman SB, Tan MP. Blood pressure lowering therapy in older people: does it really cause postural hypotension or falls? Postgrad Med 2015;127(2):186–93.

116. Mills P, Gray D, Krassioukov A. Five things to know about orthostatic hypotension and aging. J Am Geriatr Soc 2014;62(9):1822–3.

117. Butt DA, Harvey PJ. Benefits and risks of antihypertensive medications in the elderly. J Intern Med 2015;278(6):599–626.

118. Tinetti ME, Han L, Lee DS, et al. Antihypertensive medications and serious fall injuries in a nationally representative sample of older adults. JAMA Intern Med 2014;174(4):588–95.

119. Lipsitz LA, Habtemariam D, Gagnon M, et al. Reexamining the effect of antihypertensive medications on falls in old age. Hypertension 2015;66(1):183–9.

120. Lapane KL, Jesdale BM, Dubé CE, et al. Sulfonylureas and risk of falls and fractures among nursing home residents with type 2 diabetes mellitus. Diabetes Res Clin Pract 2015;109(2):411–9.

121. Lapane KL, Yang S, Brown MJ, et al. Sulfonylureas and risk of falls and fractures: a systematic review. Drugs Aging 2013;30(7):527–47.

122. Kachroo S, Kawabata H, Colilla S, et al. Association between hypoglycemia and fall-related events in type 2 diabetes mellitus: analysis of a U.S. commercial database. J Manag Care Spec Pharm 2015;21(3):243–53.

123. Signorovitch JE, Macaulay D, Diener M, et al. Hypoglycaemia and accident risk in people with type 2 diabetes mellitus treated with non-insulin antidiabetes drugs. Diabetes Obes Metab 2013;15(4):335–41.

124. Berlie HD, Garwood CL. Diabetes medications related to an increased risk of falls and fall-related morbidity in the elderly. Ann Pharmacother 2010;44(4):712–7.

125. Bohannon RW. Reference values for the timed up and go test: a descriptive meta-analysis. J Geriatr Phys Ther 2006;29(2):64–8.

126. Herman T, Giladi N, Hausdorff JM. Properties of the 'timed up and go' test: more than meets the eye. Gerontology 2011;57:203–10.

127. Viccaro LJ, Perera S, Studenski SA. Is timed up and go better than gait speed in predicting health, function and falls in older adults? J Am Geriatr Soc 2011;59:887–92.

128. MacFarlane DJ, Chou KL, Cheng YH, et al. Validity and normative data for thirty-second chair stand test in elderly community-dwelling Hong Kong Chinese. Am J Hum Biol 2006;18:418–21.

129. Rikli RE, Jones CJ. Functional fitness normative scores for community-residing older adults, ages 60-94. J Aging Phys Act 1999;7:162–81.

130. Scott V, Votova K, Scanlan A, et al. Multifactorial and functional mobility assessment tools for fall risk among older adults in community, home-support, long-term and acute care settings. Age Ageing 2007;36:130–9.

131. Guralnik JM, Simonsick EM, Ferrucci L, et al. A short physical performance battery assessing lower extremity function: association with self-reported disability and prediction of mortality and nursing home admission. J Gerontol 1994;49(2):M85–94.

132. International Pharmaceutical Federation. 2020 vision: FIP's vision, mission and strategic plan. Available at: https://www.fip.org/files/fip/strategic%20plan%20no%20annexes.pdf. Accessed June 20, 2016.

133. Centers for Medicare and Medicaid Services. Long-term care facility resident assessment instrument 3.0 user's manual, version 1.13. Available at: https://

www.cms.gov/Medicare/Quality-Initiatives-Patient-Assessment-Instruments/ NursingHomeQualityInits/Downloads/MDS-30-RAI-Manual-V113.pdf. Accessed June 20, 2016.

134. Warshany K, Sherrill CH, Cavanaugh J, et al. Medicare annual wellness visits conducted by a pharmacist in an internal medicine clinic. Am J Health Syst Pharm 2014;71(1):44–9.

Older Adult Falls in Emergency Medicine
2019 Update

Christopher R. Carpenter, MD, MSc[a],*, Amy Cameron, PA-C[b],
David A. Ganz, MD, PhD[c], Shan Liu, MD, SD[d]

KEYWORDS

- Emergency department • Accidental fall • Geriatric • Trauma • Implementation
- Emergency medical services

KEY POINTS

- Low-level falls occur in one-third of adults older than 65 each year and are a leading cause of death in developed nations.
- Injurious falls more often occur in community-dwelling older adults and usually in or around the home. Hence, prehospital providers generally represent the first-line health care professionals to manage falls and initiate innovative approaches to alleviate emergency department crowding.
- Emergency department falls research is limited in quality and quantity with continued uncertainty regarding accurate, reliable, and feasible approaches to identify high- or low-risk fallers at increased risk for recurrent falls, as well as available interventions to reduce those future falls.
- Following an episode of emergency department care, some health care systems are using a "Falls Clinic" model to expedite definitive risk assessment and fall-reduction interventions.
- Innovative approaches to assessing dynamic fall risk and fall incidence using smart phone technology are being explored.

Disclosure: The authors have nothing to disclose.
This is an update of an article that originally appeared in *Clinics in Geriatric Medicine*, Volume 34, Issue 3, August 2018.
[a] Department of Emergency Medicine and Emergency Care Research Core, Washington University in St Louis School of Medicine, Campus Box 8072, 660 South Euclid Avenue, St Louis, MO 63110, USA; [b] Department of Emergency Medicine, Massachusetts General Hospital, 55 Fruit Street, 5 Emerson, 119 C, Boston, MA 02114, USA; [c] Department of Internal Medicine Division of Geriatrics, VA Greater Los Angeles Healthcare System, David Geffen School of Medicine at UCLA, 11301 Wilshire Boulevard (11G), Los Angeles, CA 90073, USA; [d] Department of Emergency Medicine, Harvard Medical School, Massachusetts General Hospital, 5 Emerson, 119C, Boston, MA 02114, USA
* Corresponding author.
E-mail address: carpenterc@wustl.edu
; @GeriatricEDNews (C.R.C.)

Clin Geriatr Med 35 (2019) 205–219
https://doi.org/10.1016/j.cger.2019.01.009
0749-0690/19/© 2019 Elsevier Inc. All rights reserved.

EPIDEMIOLOGY OF FALLS

Aging populations worldwide are reshaping the epidemiology of trauma.[1] Older persons, generally described as aged 65 or older, comprise approximately one-fourth of trauma admissions, and trauma-related injuries are the fifth leading cause of death in the United States with 29,668 fall deaths in 2016.[2] Aging trauma victims have twice the mortality of younger patients when adjusted for Injury Severity Score, but even minor trauma mechanisms like ground-level falls can precipitate rapid functional decline, preventable emergency department recidivism, and diminished quality of life. In fact, approximately one-third of older fall patients discharged from the emergency department experience one of these outcomes at 3 months.[3] Between 36% and 50% of patients have an adverse event, such as a recurrent fall, emergency department revisit, or death within 1 year after a fall.[4,5] The challenge for health care providers is to identify which emergency department patients will suffer short-term adverse outcomes, and to develop feasible, widely available interventions to reduce these sequelae.[6] Prehospital, emergency department, and trauma services continue to adapt in response to this evolving epidemiology of trauma.[7]

Definitions for falls vary across studies, but recently the Prevention of Falls Network Europe (ProFaNE) has become one widely accepted descriptor as "an unexpected event in which the participants come to rest on the ground, floor, or lower level."[8] The prevalence of falls is largely derived from single-center retrospective studies or secondary analyses of administrative databases, both of which may simultaneously underestimate the scope of fall injuries and overestimate the observed value of diagnostic and therapeutic interventions.[9] However, algorithmic approaches to improve the value of Medicare data are now under way,[10] as well as chart review methods that augment International al Classification of Diseases, Ninth Revision codes with the patient's chief complaint.[11] At least 1 fall occurs each year in approximately one-third of *community-dwelling* individuals older than 65, increasing to 50% of those older than 80.[12–14] Among those living at home, falls usually occur in and around the home with 20% causing potentially life-threatening injuries.

Frailty is an important predictor of falls, but accurate measures of vulnerability among older adults in emergency department settings do not exist.[14,15] Similarly, existing constructs of "frailty" fail to accurately identify subsets of *nursing home* residents at increased risk for falls.[16] However, injurious falls presenting to emergency department trauma units are more commonly *community-dwelling* individuals.[17] Once patients are hospitalized, 3 to 5 inpatient falls per 1000 patient-days occur across medical, neurologic, and surgical populations with 2% resulting in fractures.[18] Geography is another factor in assessing the sequelae of falls. Rural fall victims are less likely to be hospitalized, have a shorter duration of hospital length of stay, and demonstrate higher 1-month readmission rates and mortality.[19] In the United States, direct medical costs associated with falls totaled $616 million for fatal and $30 billion for nonfatal injurious falls in 2012, with significant variability between states.[20,21] As fall-related hospitalizations and associated costs continue rising, emergency department identification of older adults at higher risk for fall-related injuries will become increasingly relevant. By comparison, the cost of annual cancer care represents a similar economic burden, and emergency department physicians accept a role in preventing cancer via smoking-cessation efforts.[22] Nonetheless, emergency department fall interventions have yet to demonstrate cost-effectiveness, so quantifying the benefits and harms of fall-prevention strategies remains an unmet challenge.[23,24] This review focuses on prehospital and emergency department fall-risk screening and interventions and real-world barriers to implementation of these concepts, while exploring evolving approaches to management, such as post–emergency department falls clinics and technological approaches to monitor falls and fall risk factors.

PREHOSPITAL FALL RISK ASSESSMENT AND PREVENTIVE INTERVENTIONS

Emergency medical services (EMS) report a threefold increase in fall-related calls between 2007 and 2017.[25] The traditional scoop and run paradigm has shifted to a more evaluative, patient-centered process that empowers paramedics and paramedic extenders to assess intrinsic and extrinsic risks for future falls, because a subset of patients are heavy EMS users who infrequently require transportation.[26,27] Emergency department and primary care providers often are not aware of EMS fall evaluations when patients are not transported to the hospital. Reducing injurious falls will require more efficient communication among various downstream providers, patients, and families. Although pain or altered functional status are associated with transportation to the emergency department, EMS calls from personal alarm devices are less likely to be associated with the patient being transported.[28] When fall victims are not transported to the emergency department, they may be referred to a "Falls Clinic" (discussed later) or provided information about other fall-prevention services. Reducing recurrent injurious falls among patients in either prehospital or emergency department settings depends on reliable patient follow-up and often patient adherence to behavioral changes such as physical therapy, as well as identification of the subset of fall victims most likely to benefit from preventive interventions.

EMS research thus far has demonstrated inconsistent fall-prevention benefits and no effect on reducing injurious falls.[29] One British EMS protocol trained prehospital providers to use an algorithm assessing fall risk and refer appropriate fallers who were not transported to the emergency department to a "Fall Clinic." This intervention reduced future emergency calls, but did not decrease or increase short-term injury risk and had a mean cost of $23 per patient.[30]

Multiple issues likely underlie the failure of EMS interventions to consistently reduce fall-related injuries. First, each region's EMS system represents a unique fiefdom with variable institutional interest in healthy aging or falls prevention buried within a constellation of competing priorities. Adapting EMS educational priorities with the guidance of a geriatric emergency medicine opinion leader has successfully overcome this inertia in some settings.[31] Second, reliably accurate, widely accepted, and routinely available EMS protocols to risk-stratify and intervene on fall victims do not exist.[29] The disappointing results of prior research may indicate selection of the patients less likely to benefit from specific interventions, because fall victims have a heterogeneous mixture of risk factors and comorbid illness burden. Third, referral to a "Falls Clinic" or to primary care is a black box intervention dependent on patient compliance and effectiveness of the subsequent fall-reduction interventions, as is discussed later.

EMERGENCY DEPARTMENT AND POST–EMERGENCY DEPARTMENT FALL RISK ASSESSMENT AND INTERVENTIONS

Unfortunately, the subset of fall victims who are transported by EMS (or arrive by other transportation) to the emergency department do not often receive guidelines-directed care.[32,33] Multiple emergency medicine and geriatrics professional societies have endorsed fall management guidelines (**Fig. 1**),[34] yet these recommendations remain largely untested and unavailable for many emergency department settings. In resource-strained emergency department settings, it is neither fiscally viable nor feasible to label every older adult as high risk for emergency department or post-discharge falls. Yet relative to the injury burden falls represent, there is a paucity of

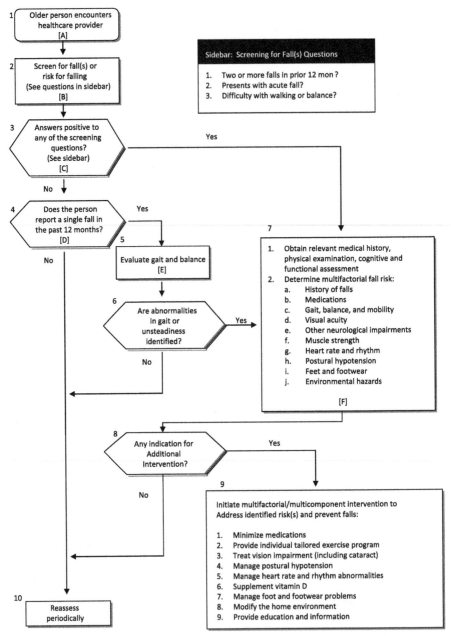

Fig. 1. American Geriatric Society/British Geriatric Society Guidelines to prevent falls in community-residing elderly. mon, months. (*From* Panel on Prevention of Falls in Older Persons, American Geriatrics Society, British Geriatrics Society. Summary of the updated American Geriatrics Society/British Geriatrics Society clinical practice guideline for prevention of falls in older persons. J Am Geriatr Soc 2011;59(1):150; with permission.)

emergency department research to develop instruments and predictors to distinguish high-risk from non–high-risk future fallers.[13] Triage nurses also evaluate fall risk, which can be a useful process for emergency department providers and inpatient services if effectively communicated between providers.[35]

Surprisingly, objective functional assessments like Get Up and Go have not accurately predicted future fall risk in emergency department patients.[36–39] This inaccuracy may reflect patient selection rather than test properties, because the Timed Up and Go Test is more accurate in lower functioning older adults than in healthier community-dwelling individuals.[40] Emergency medicine nursing studies focus primarily on falls within the emergency department, which are not comparable with post–emergency department fall instruments or interventions. In addition, nursing studies of fall instruments do not provide quantitative accuracy results for comparison with other screening instruments.[41,42] Ongoing efforts to derive, validate, and evaluate the impact of fall-risk instruments have proven challenging because of the large number of intrinsic and extrinsic factors associated with older adult falls and fall-related injuries (**Fig. 2**). Nonetheless, brief post–emergency department fall-risk screening instruments exist that seem to distinguish low-risk from higher-risk emergency department patients (**Box 1**).[13]

The most recent Cochrane review of multifactorial interventions to reduce falls in community-dwelling older adults included 62 trials, but only 1 based in the emergency department.[43] Distinguishing emergency department studies from others is pertinent because interventions to reduce fall-related injuries generally rely on personnel, equipment, and resources that are unavailable in most contemporary emergency departments.[12] For example, the Prevention of Falls in the Elderly Trial (PROFET) randomized cognitively intact patients older than 65 following an emergency department falls-related visit to either routine care or to a detailed collaborative evaluation by a geriatrician and occupational therapist within 1 week of emergency department discharge. The comprehensive geriatric evaluation assessed visual acuity, balance, affect, mental status, and postural hypotension in a "day clinic," with appropriate referrals based on these findings.[44] Few emergency departments have access to a "day clinic," geriatrician, or occupational therapist and perhaps not surprisingly the PROFET results have not been replicated. Another recent emergency department randomized controlled trial not included in the Cochrane review also found that individualized multifactorial interventions failed to reduce falls rates at 1 year.[45]

However, factors associated with suboptimal fall-related emergency department outcomes are becoming clearer. Poverty, lack of supplemental insurance, and extremity injuries are predictors of subsequent hospital admission for older adults after discharge from the emergency department following blunt trauma.[46] Telephone follow-up for emergency department fall patients is feasible and may reduce subsequent falls.[47] On the other hand, although some medications are associated with increased fall risk, de-prescribing these medications in emergency department patients does not consistently reduce subsequent fall risk within a year.[48] One limitation of emergency department de-prescribing is that primary care providers often re-start these same medications.

ONLINE EMERGENCY DEPARTMENT FALL RESOURCES

Emergency department providers rely on outpatient fall resources for comprehensive risk assessment and definitive prevention interventions. Identifying these resources real-time during a clinical shift is challenging because no central repository exists. Web-based resources from "fall clinics" include Johns Hopkins, University of

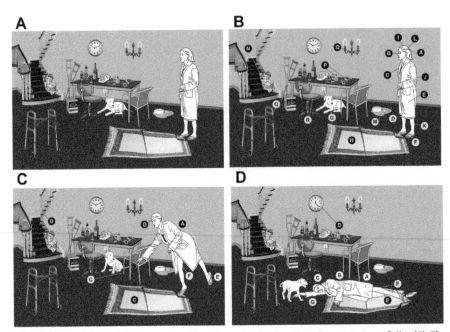

Fig. 2. (*A*) Understanding geriatric fall risks and factors related to injurious falls. (*B*) The older adult before a fall and illustrates the intrinsic (physiological attributes of the individual) and extrinsic (environmental surroundings) that can be related to a fall. Some of these factors are evidence-based from epidemiological studies (denoted with "*"), whereas others are recognized by the clinician authors of this review. These risk factors include the following: (A) disequilibrium*; (B) visual deficits; (C) dysrhythmia, orthostatic hypotension; (D) degenerative joint disease and rheumatic disease*; (E) loose-fitting clothing; (F) poorly fitting footwear or foot sores; (G) pets; (H) rugs or loose mats; (I) dementia, Parkinson Disease*; (J) malnutrition; (K) deconditioning, frailty, muscle wasting; (L) preexisting stroke or other motor deficit*; (M) slippery surface; (N) stairs with clutter and urinary incontinence* pads; (O) walker or crutches; (P) medications (sedatives),* alcohol, also note the falls alert device (not worn) and the eyeglasses; (Q) inadequate lighting; (R) transfers from sitting to standing (in this illustration with a chair that is not stable). (*C*) Intrinsic and extrinsic factors that render older adults more likely to suffer a fall than a near-fall. Whereas younger populations sometimes suffer near-falls, they rarely fall to the ground and when they do the kinetic energy of the fall is usually disrupted by a variety of adaptive protection responses that are slowed, diminished, or absent in frail older persons. These factors include the following: (A) impaired reflexes to ease fall, (B) lack of handrails, (C) cluttered furniture, (D) diminished awareness of falling, (E) impaired proprioception, and (F) diminished core body strength. (*D*) The physiologic, pharmacologic, anatomic, and environmental factors that increase the probability of the primary fall injury severity for the mechanism and energy of a fall becoming more pronounced and for secondary injuries to ensue. (A) Osteoporosis = fractures with minor trauma, (B) spinal cord stenosis and cervical spine degenerative disc disease = spinal cord contusion (anterior cord syndrome), (C) cerebral wasting = subdural hematoma, (D) medications (anticoagulants, antiplatelet agents) = increased risk of intracranial (and other) bleeding (note the time on the clock as it compares with **Fig. 2**C), (E) muscle wasting = inability to rise and "long waiting times on the ground," (F) diminished body fat/padding = more force to brittle bones, (G) frail skin = tears and lacerations. (*Image* created by Christopher Carpenter MD, MSc and Michael Malone, MD. Reproduced with permission of Aurora Health Care, Inc., Milwaukee, WI.)

Box 1
Emergency department fall risk stratification instruments

Carpenter[36]
1. Presence of nonhealing foot sore?
2. Any fall in past 12 months?
3. Inability to cut own toenails?
4. Self-reported depression?

Interpretation greater than 1 "yes" responses is a community-dwelling older adult at increased risk for falls.

Tiedemann[37]
1. Two or more falls in the past year? (2 points)
2. Take 6 or more medications? (1 point)

Interpretation Score >2 = older adult at increased risk for falls.

Wisconsin Medicine, Live Long Walk Strong at Spaulding Rehabilitation Center in Cambridge, Massachusetts, and The University of Vermont Medical Center. **Table 1** provides a nonexhaustive list of Web addresses for representative "fall clinics." The Johns Hopkins "falls clinic" evaluation includes a screening questionnaire, physical therapy and occupational therapy assessment, comprehensive evaluation, and referrals to specialist physician, if needed. The Live Long Walk Strong program evaluates patients sent to the clinic by their primary care provider. As previously noted, the American College of Emergency Physicians' (ACEP) Geriatric Emergency Department Guidelines outlines an extensive workup for fall patients.[34] ACEP also created the *7 Step Fall Challenge*, a 7-minute video available on YouTube that clinicians can share with emergency department patients to educate them on fall risk and prevention. In addition, Free Open Access Medical Education (FOAMed) resources increasingly

---

Table 1
Online fall resources

	Fall Clinics
Johns Hopkins	(http://www.hopkinsmedicine.org/physical_medicine_rehabilitation/services/programs/falls-prevention.html)
University of Wisconsin	(http://www.fammed.wisc.edu/northeast-clinic-takes-steps-prevent-elderly-falls/),
Live Long Walk Strong	(http://spauldingrehab.org/conditions-and-treatments/live-long-walk-strong),
University of Vermont Medical Center	(https://www.uvmhealth.org/medcenter/pages/Departments-and-Programs/Fall-Prevention.aspx).
	Emergency Medicine Cases
ACEP 7 Step Fall Challenge	(https://www.youtube.com/watch?v=-ehHhdoJ2k8
FOAMed	(https://emergencymedicinecases.com/episode-34-geriatric-emergency-medicine/)
The Skeptics Guide to Emergency Medicine	http://thesgem.com/2014/10/sgem89-preventing-falling-to-pieces/
Geri-EM	https://geri-em.com/
GEMCAST	https://gempodcast.com/2017/03/13/ems-preventing-falls/#more-459

highlight fall management challenges, including EM Cases and Skeptics Guide to Emergency Medicine. Geri-EM is an interactive e-learning Web site focused on geriatric emergencies and including free continuing medical education with topics ranging from falls to end-of-life issues.

POST–EMERGENCY DEPARTMENT FALLS CLINIC

Access to falls clinics in the United States is inconsistent, but health outcomes researchers continue to explore the key attributes and efficacy of these outpatient resources. In the Netherlands, there are 23 fall clinics. Screening emergency department and primary care patients with the CAREFALL Triage Instrument suggests that on average patients referred to a fall clinic from the emergency department have more fall risk factors than do those referred by primary care. More importantly, patients referred from an emergency department have risk factors different from those referred from primary care, which may influence the impact of interventions.[49]

Linking high-risk fall patients in the emergency department with appropriate outpatient resources is challenging. Simply distributing information about local falls prevention programs is unlikely to reduce fall rates or injuries.[50] In addition, although emergency department patients may report willingness to follow-up with a falls clinic, actual compliance rates are often quite low.[51] Patients in a pilot fall-prevention referral study report low compliance secondary to transportation barriers, disinterest, and lack of sufficient motivation (Shan Liu, MD, SD, personal communication, 2019). Reducing recurrent falls will also depend on identifying and overcoming barriers to patient follow-up. Shared decision making and fall-specific patient aids may be one approach to improving patient compliance with fall-reduction interventions.[52]

KNOWLEDGE TRANSLATION BARRIERS

Knowledge translation begins with definitive research evidence. One immediate challenge for emergency medicine falls intervention is that much of the evidence regarding risk assessment and intervention has been developed for primary care doctors (for example, one guideline from the American Geriatrics Society, one from Stopping Elderly Accidents Death and Injuries, and another from the US Preventive Services Task Force).[53–55] No single, well-accepted, simple test or intervention like a troponin level or a coronary catheterization exists for falls. Instead, fall risk assessments are complex, multifactorial endeavors that can consume 10 to 15 minutes. The vast majority of emergency department clinicians are unwilling to spend more than 5 minutes on fall risk assessment and intervention (Shan Liu, MD, SD, personal communication, 2019). In addition, emergency department fall patients often have acute injuries, weakness, delirium, or other chief complaints that make using commonly cited risk assessment instruments challenging.[53] In multiple studies, most emergency department fall patients are unable to comply with functional tests like the Timed Get up and Go (Shan Liu, MD, SD, personal communication, 2019).[36] The following important unanswered questions remain:

1. Which patients should undergo a risk assessment?
2. What functional tests should be conducted, if any?
3. What interventions are feasible in the emergency department?

Most emergency department clinicians cannot identify the approximate proportion of community-dwelling elderly patients who fall annually. Effective shared decision making relies on informed health care providers,[56] but two-thirds of emergency department clinicians are unfamiliar with ACEP fall-prevention guidelines.[34] Although

80% of respondents in one survey believe it is very important for them to prevent recurrent falls among elderly emergency department patients, 46% would spend less than 2 minutes to do so. Most (87%) providers believe that there is not enough time to implement geriatric falls prevention in the emergency department. There is a need to do more training to general emergency department providers about fall risk factors and risk prevention (Shan Liu, MD, SD, personal communication, 2019), but education alone is unlikely to sustainably improve emergency department falls management.[33] Alternatively, these data may necessitate creative interventions that do not depend on emergency department providers, such as a mobile falls assessment team, geriatric/physical therapy consults in the emergency department, or outside-the-box interventions such as incentives for emergency department providers who implement fall-prevention interventions.

Which older adults should emergency department providers evaluate for fall risk? One approach would be to evaluate all geriatric adults' fall risk, though it is unlikely that most emergency department providers would screen all geriatric patients who come to the emergency department given the competing priorities of other patients. A more tangible approach would focus on recent fallers (within the past 2–4 weeks) because their chief complaint likely is related to their fall; the emergency department visit as a sentinel event could serve as an opportune teachable moment for high-risk patients.[57] Another option is to only intervene on fall patients who are discharged, because 75% of patients are discharged and in-hospital teams can more easily consult physical therapy or design more time-intensive fall-prevention programs. Ethical and pragmatic issues with delirium or nursing home patients also exist. These vulnerable subsets are more likely to be at risk of recurrent falls, but also may be the most difficult to prevent recurrent falls secondary to underlying frailty, disease burden, and cognitive impairment. For example, one multifactorial intervention in cognitively impaired emergency department patients was ineffective.[58]

Unfortunately, determining which patients to screen, when to screen them, and who is best suited to screen them is only the first issue. An even more challenging question is what type of interventions are effective, available, and feasible for emergency department fall patients and their health care providers? Similarly, emergency department physicians will be hesitant to change sleep, depression, anxiety, and cardiovascular medications that specialists and primary care physicians have prescribed. However, the ongoing opioid epidemic is refocusing attention on analgesic prescribing and falls.[59] Practically speaking, emergency department physicians are likely only to implement interventions that are streamlined and highly effective in reducing recurrent falls. One challenge is the need to create fall programs in the emergency department that follow implementation science principles and/or quality improvement strategies to maximize successful outcomes.[53,60,61]

Another challenge is that it takes a village to be successful at managing an individual's fall risk.[62] Family members, patients, EMS, and emergency department providers who often are the first clinicians to see someone after a fall, primary care doctors, physical therapists, case managers, and geriatricians all have a stake in fall management. For example, physical therapy services in the emergency department are associated with fewer revisits up to 2 months.[63] Multidisciplinary hip fracture pathways can reduce emergency department and hospital length of stay, while also reducing inpatient complications.[64] However, rarely are transdisciplinary falls experts and stakeholders at the same national/international meetings or institutional Grand Rounds to discuss lessons learned or to share stories of success. Although interventions likely need to be tailored to the local environment, such conferences would likely be invaluable to encourage support, innovation, collaboration, and inspiration.

FUTURE OF EMERGENCY DEPARTMENT FALLS MANAGEMENT

Technology-based interventions have been used in a wide range of fall-prevention efforts, including diagnosing and managing fall risk, improving intervention adherence, and fall detection.[65] For example, a feasibility study using calcaneal ultrasound as one quantitative predictor of falls was recently published.[66] Other devices (ie, mobile phone–based systems) have many advantages, namely their popularity, decreasing costs, and portability.[67] Most smartphones also integrate all the required elements to develop autonomous and self-sufficient fall-detection applications.

Technology also has been seen as a means to help patients self-assess their risk of falling, which can potentially save money if patients do not need to do initial screening with a clinician.[65] This may be key to reducing costs as well as improving quality of care.[65] The "Aachen Fall Prevention App" (AFPA) is the first reported mobile health application that empowers older patients (>50 years) to self-assess and monitor their fall risk.[68] This was created by German providers from the Department of Orthopedic Trauma. The self-assessment consists of 3 steps based on the "Aachen Fall Prevention Scale."[69] The first step consists of patients answering 10 yes-no questions. The second step consists of a 10-second test of patients standing, which is considered positive if there is compensatory movement. A final step asks patients to rate their subjective fall risk on a 10-point Likert scale adjusted to the results of the first 2 steps. The app was created to allow patients to independently monitor their individual fall risk as well as collect data about how a patient-centered mobile health application could be used in the field. From December 2015 to December 2016, 197 people downloaded the AFPA, of which 79 people were ultimately analyzed after other subjects were excluded or did not share their data. Preliminary data showed a significant positive correlation between objective fall risk and the self-assessment data obtained by the AFPA.[68] Although the AFPA currently is available only in German, it represents a first promising step in raising older adults' awareness of their fall risk and could be a tool that is adapted for the emergency department population.

Early detection of falls is also important, as long waiting times on the ground increase the risk of hospitalization and death.[70] Traditionally, fall alert systems depend on the older adult pushing a button and communicating with a central operating system. These systems may be less useful if the range of the device is restricted to the home or if the person cannot push the button (eg, if he or she is unconscious).[71] Hence, using the accelerometer feature in today's smart phones, which older adults can easily carry, represents a promising new technology. There is a plethora of work being conducted to develop smartphone-based fall-detection systems.[67] False negatives (fall has occurred but device did not recognize a fall) might be problematic using smartphones and the rate of missed falls will depend on the type of falls (forward vs lateral vs backward falls), type of algorithm used to determine if a fall has occurred, and where the smartphone is placed (waist vs thigh). The percentage of false negatives ranges from (1.2–29.9) depending on the type of fall and the different application algorithms. False-positive (no fall occurred but device alarms as if a fall did happen) rates range from 5.9% to 21.9% depending on the various algorithms. No algorithm had an efficiency higher than 95% or 90% to avoid false positives and false negatives, respectively.[67] Biomedical engineers are now assessing the combined ability of smartphone and smart-watches to detect falls. Vilarinho and colleagues[71] found that together, the smartphone/smart-watch could correctly identify 63% of falls. The Apple Watch Series 4 can detect falls and call EMS if a faller does not respond or agrees with the call.

Passive monitoring systems also exist and can be used in assisted living facilities to monitor falls. Patel and Gunnarsson[72] described a passive monitoring system that uses advanced motion sensor technology that learns the daily patterns of community residents in a senior home and sends alerts when abnormal events occur. Their study compared falls, hospitalizations, and resident attrition between one facility that adopted the monitoring system and a control facility over a 12-month period. Monitoring reduced falls and improved resident retention compared with the control group.[72]

SUMMARY

Geriatric falls are both frequent and associated with rapid functional decline, preventable emergency department recidivism, diminished quality of life, and mortality. EMS is increasingly assessing fall patients in their home environments and in some settings referring patients to fall clinics without transporting them to the emergency department. However, EMS interventions have thus far not been able to demonstrate decreased risk of fall-related injuries. Emergency medicine and geriatric professional societies have endorsed fall management guidelines, but standard emergency department care often fails to adhere to these recommendations. Researchers using post–emergency department evaluations by a geriatrician and physical therapist have successfully decreased recurrent falls among emergency department fall patients, but await replication in other settings. Most emergency departments lack access to fall clinics or other intra–emergency department or post–emergency department fall-prevention resources, but multiple open access educational resources for social workers, nurses, and physicians are now available. Fall interventions are often multifactorial, complicated, and time-consuming, making it challenging to create a streamlined assessment and prevention of fall algorithm for emergency department patients. Survey data indicate that educating emergency department clinicians on fall epidemiology and available resources is a priority. Furthermore, emergency department clinicians are unwilling to spend more than 5 minutes on fall risk assessment and intervention, so implementation science is needed to align fall patients' needs with contemporary emergency care. In the future, emergency department falls management may be assisted with the use of technology to help assess patient fall risk and facilitate more timely acute and preventive interventions.

ACKNOWLEDGMENTS

The authors wish to thank Mr. Brian J. Miller and Dr. Michael Malone from Aurora Health Care for their contributions in developing **Figure 2** of this article.

REFERENCES

1. Carpenter CR, Rosen PI. Trauma in the geriatric patient. In: Mattu A, Grossman SA, Rosen PI, et al, editors. Geriatric emergencies: a discussion-based review. Oxford (United Kingdom): Wiley-Blackwell; 2016. p. 280–303.

2. Burns E, Kakara R. Deaths from falls among persons aged ≥65 years - United States, 2007-2016. MMWR Morb Wkly Rep 2018;67(18):509–14.

3. Sirois MJ, Emond M, Ouellet MC, et al. Cumulative incidence of functional decline following minor injuries in previously independent older Canadian emergency department patients. J Am Geriatr Soc 2013;61(10):1661–8.

4. Liu SW, Obermeyer Z, Chang Y, et al. Frequency of ED revisits and death among older adults after a fall. Am J Emerg Med 2015;33(8):1012–8.

5. Sri-On J, Tirrell GP, Bean JF, et al. Revisit, subsequent hospitalization, recurrent fall, and death within 6 months after a fall among elderly emergency department patients. Ann Emerg Med 2017;70(4):516–21.e2.

6. Carpenter CR. Deteriorating functional status in older adults after emergency department evaluation of minor trauma-opportunities and pragmatic challenges. J Am Geriatr Soc 2013;61(10):1806–7.

7. Carpenter CR, Arendts G, Hullick C, et al. Major trauma in the older patient: evolving trauma care beyond management of bumps and bruises. Emerg Med Australas 2017;29(4):450–5.

8. Lamb SE, Jørstad-Stein EC, Hauer K, et al. Development of a common outcome data set for fall injury prevention trials: the prevention of Falls Network Europe consensus. J Am Geriatr Soc 2005;53(9):1618–22.

9. Hoffman JR, Carpenter CR. Guarding against overtesting, overdiagnosis, and overtreatment of older adults: thinking beyond imaging and injuries to weigh harms and benefits. J Am Geriatr Soc 2017;65(5):903–5.

10. Kim SB, Zingmond DS, Keeler EB, et al. Development of an algorithm to identify fall-related injuries and costs in Medicare data. Inj Epidemiol 2016;3(1):1.

11. Patterson BW, Smith MA, Repplinger MD, et al. Using chief complaint in addition to diagnosis codes to identify falls in the emergency department. J Am Geriatr Soc 2017;65(9):E135–40.

12. Carpenter CR. Falls and fall prevention in the elderly. In: Kahn JH, Magauran BG, Olshaker JS, editors. Geriatric emergency medicine principles and practice. Cambridge (United Kingdom): Cambridge University Press; 2014. p. 343–50.

13. Carpenter CR, Avidan MS, Wildes T, et al. Predicting community-dwelling older adult falls following an episode of emergency department care: a systematic review. Acad Emerg Med 2014;21(10):1069–82.

14. Carpenter CR, Shelton E, Fowler S, et al. Risk factors and screening instruments to predict adverse outcomes for undifferentiated older emergency department patients: a systematic review and meta-analysis. Acad Emerg Med 2015;22(1):1–21.

15. Bandeen-Roche K, Seplaki CL, Huang J, et al. Frailty in older adults: a nationally representative profile in the United States. J Gerontol A Biol Sci Med Sci 2015;70(11):1427–34.

16. Buckinx F, Croisier JL, Reginster JY, et al. Prediction of the incidence of falls and deaths among elderly nursing home residents: the SENIOR study. J Am Med Dir Assoc 2018;19(1):18–24.

17. Evans D, Pester J, Vera L, et al. Elderly fall patients triaged to the trauma bay: age, injury patterns, and mortality risk. Am J Emerg Med 2015;33(11):1635–8.

18. Lake ET, Shang J, Klaus S, et al. Patient falls: association with hospital Magnet status and nursing unit staffing. Res Nurs Health 2010;33(5):413–25.

19. Sukumar DW, Harvey LA, Mitchell RJ, et al. The impact of geographical location on trends in hospitalisation rates and outcomes for fall-related injuries in older people. Aust N Z J Public Health 2016;40(4):342–8.

20. Burns ER, Stevens JA, Lee R. The direct costs of fatal and non-fatal falls among older adults - United States. J Safety Res 2016;58:99–103.

21. Haddad YK, Bergen G, Florence CS. Estimating the economic burden related to older adult falls by state. J Public Health Manag Pract 2019;25(2):E17–24.

22. Platts-Mills T. Emergency care providers and falls in the elderly: are we ready for primary prevention? Emergencias 2018;30(4):221–3.

23. Harper KJ, Arendts G, Geelhoed EA, et al. Cost analysis of a brief intervention for the prevention of falls after discharge from an emergency department. J Eval Clin Pract 2018. [Epub ahead of print].

24. Matchar DB, Eom K, Duncan PW, et al. A cost-effectiveness analysis of a randomized control trial of a tailored, multifactorial program to prevent falls among the community-dwelling elderly. Arch Phys Med Rehabil 2018;100(1):1–8.

25. Quatman CE, Mondor M, Halweg J, et al. Ten years of EMS fall calls in a community: an opportunity for injury prevention strategies. Geriatr Orthop Surg Rehabil 2018;9. 2151459318783453.

26. Munjal KG, Shastry S, Loo GT, et al. Patient perspectives on EMS alternate destination models. Prehosp Emerg Care 2016;20(6):705–11.

27. Quatman CE, Anderson JP, Mondor M, et al. Frequent 911 fall calls in older adults: opportunity for injury prevention strategies. J Am Geriatr Soc 2018; 66(9):1737–43.

28. Simpson PM, Bendall JC, Toson B, et al. Predictors of nontransport of older fallers who receive ambulance care. Prehosp Emerg Care 2014;18(3):342–9.

29. Zozula A, Carpenter CR, Lipsey K, et al. Prehospital emergency services screening and referral to reduce falls in community-dwelling older adults: a systematic review. Emerg Med J 2016;33(5):345–50.

30. Snooks HA, Anthony R, Chatters R, et al. Support and Assessment for Fall Emergency Referrals (SAFER) 2: a cluster randomised trial and systematic review of clinical effectiveness and cost-effectiveness of new protocols for emergency ambulance paramedics to assess older people following a fall with referral to community-based care when appropriate. Health Technol Assess 2017;21(13): 1–218.

31. Shah MN, Caprio TV, Swanson P, et al. A novel emergency medical services-based program to identify and assist older adults in a rural community. J Am Geriatr Soc 2010;58(11):2205–11.

32. Tirrell G, Sri-on J, Lipsitz LA, et al. Evaluation of older adult patients with falls in the emergency department: discordance with national guidelines. Acad Emerg Med 2015;22(4):461–7.

33. McEwan H, Baker R, Armstrong N, et al. A qualitative study of the determinants of adherence to NICE falls guideline in managing older fallers attending an emergency department. Int J Emerg Med 2018;11(1):33.

34. Rosenberg M, Carpenter CR, Bromley M, et al. Geriatric emergency department guidelines. Ann Emerg Med 2014;63(5):e7–25.

35. Southerland LT, Slattery L, Rosenthal JA, et al. Are triage questions sufficient to assign fall risk precautions in the ED? Am J Emerg Med 2017;35(2):329–32.

36. Carpenter CR, Scheatzle MD, D'Antonio JA, et al. Identification of fall risk factors in older adult emergency department patients. Acad Emerg Med 2009;16(3): 211–9.

37. Tiedemann A, Sherrington C, Orr T, et al. Identifying older people at high risk of future falls: development and validation of a screening tool for use in emergency departments. Emerg Med J 2013;30(11):918–22.

38. Eagles D, Yadav K, Perry JJ, et al. Mobility assessments of geriatric emergency department patients: a systematic review. CJEM 2017;20(3):353–61.

39. Chow RB, Lee A, Kane BG, et al. Effectiveness of the "timed up and go" (TUG) and the chair test as screening tools for geriatric fall risk assessment in the ED. Am J Emerg Med 2018. [Epub ahead of print].

40. Schoene D, Wu SM, Mikolaizak AS, et al. Discriminative ability and predictive validity of the timed up and go test in identifying older people who fall: systematic review and meta-analysis. J Am Geriatr Soc 2013;61(2):202–8.

41. Scott RA, Oman KS, Flarity K, et al. Above, beyond, and over the side rails: evaluating the new memorial emergency department fall-risk-assessment tool. J Emerg Nurs 2018;44(5):483–90.

42. Amesz S. Above, beyond, and over the side rails: evaluating the new memorial emergency department fall-risk-assessment tool. J Emerg Nurs 2018;44(5):444.

43. Hopewell S, Adedire O, Copsey BJ, et al. Multifactorial and multiple component interventions for preventing falls in older people living in the community. Cochrane Database Syst Rev 2018;(7):CD012221.

44. Close J, Ellis M, Hooper R, et al. Prevention of falls in the elderly trial (PROFET): a randomised controlled trial. Lancet 1999;353(9147):93–7.

45. Tan PJ, Khoo EM, Chinna K, et al. Individually-tailored multifactorial intervention to reduce falls in the Malaysian Falls Assessment and Intervention Trial (MyFAIT): a randomized controlled trial. PLoS One 2018;13(8):e0199219.

46. Earl-Royal EC, Kaufman EJ, Hanlon AL, et al. Factors associated with hospital admission after an emergency department treat and release visit for older adults with injuries. Am J Emerg Med 2017;35(9):1252–7.

47. Phelan EA, Pence M, Williams B, et al. Telephone care management of fall risk: a feasibility study. Am J Prev Med 2017;52(3S3):S290–4.

48. Boyé ND, Van der Velde N, de Vries OJ, et al. Effectiveness of medication withdrawal in older fallers: results from the Improving Medication Prescribing to reduce Risk Of FALLs (IMPROveFALL) trial. Age Ageing 2017;46(1):142–6.

49. Schoon Y, Hoogsteen-Ossewaarde ME, Scheffer AC, et al. Comparison of different strategies of referral to a fall clinic: how to achieve an optimal casemix? J Nutr Health Aging 2011;15(2):140–5.

50. Baraff LJ, Lee TJ, Kader S, et al. Effect of a practice guideline on the process of emergency department care of falls in elder patients. Acad Emerg Med 1999; 6(12):1216–23.

51. Shankar KN, Treadway NJ, Taylor AA, et al. Older adult falls prevention behaviors 60 days post-discharge from an urban emergency department after treatment for a fall. Inj Epidemiol 2017;4(1):18.

52. Hogan TM, Richmond NL, Carpenter CR, et al. Shared decision making to improve the emergency care of older adults: a research agenda. Acad Emerg Med 2016;23(12):1386–93.

53. Carpenter CR, Lo AX. Falling behind? Understanding implementation science in future emergency department management strategies for geriatric fall prevention. Acad Emerg Med 2015;22(4):478–80.

54. Panel on Prevention of Falls in Older Persons, American Geriatrics Society and British Geriatrics Society. Summary of the updated American Geriatrics Society/British Geriatrics Society clinical practice guideline for prevention of falls in older persons. J Am Geriatr Soc 2011;59(1):148–57.

55. Guirguis-Blake JM, Michael YL, Perdue LA, et al. Interventions to prevent falls in older adults: updated evidence report and systematic review for the US Preventive Services Task Force. JAMA 2018;319(16):1705–16.

56. Hess EP, Grudzen CR, Thomson R, et al. Shared decision-making in the Emergency Department: respecting patient autonomy when seconds count. Acad Emerg Med 2015;22(7):856–64.

57. Tinetti ME, Baker DI, McAvay G, et al. A multifactorial intervention to reduce the risk of falling among elderly people living in the community. N Engl J Med 1994; 331(13):821–7.

58. Shaw FE, Bond J, Richardson DA, et al. Multifactorial intervention after a fall in older people with cognitive impairment and dementia presenting to the accident and emergency department: randomised controlled trial. BMJ 2003;326(7380): 73.

59. Daoust R, Paquet J, Moore L, et al. Recent opioid use and fall-related injury among older patients with trauma. CMAJ 2018;190(16):E500–6.

60. Neta G, Glasgow RE, Carpenter CR, et al. A framework for enhancing the value of research for dissemination and implementation. Am J Public Health 2015;105(1): 49–57.

61. Stoeckle A, Iseler JI, Havey R, et al. Catching quality before it falls: preventing falls and injuries in the adult emergency department. J Emerg Nurs 2018. [Epub ahead of print].

62. Ganz DA, Alkema GE, Wu S. It takes a village to prevent falls: reconceptualizing fall prevention and management for older adults. Inj Prev 2008;14(4):266–71.

63. Lesser A, Israni J, Kent T, et al. Association between physical therapy in the Emergency Department and Emergency Department revisits for older adult fallers: a nationally representative analysis. J Am Geriatr Soc 2018;66(1): 2205–12.

64. Wallace R, Angus LDG, Munnanqi S, et al. Improved outcomes following implementation of a multidisciplinary care pathway for elderly hip fractures. Aging Clin Exp Res 2019;31(2):273–8.

65. Hamm J, Money AG, Atwal A, et al. Fall prevention intervention technologies: a conceptual framework and survey of the state of the art. J Biomed Inform 2016;59:319–45.

66. Ou LC, Chang YF, Chang CS, et al. Epidemiological survey of the feasibility of broadband ultrasound attenuation measured using calcaneal quantitative ultrasound to predict the incidence of falls in the middle aged and elderly. BMJ Open 2017;7(1):e013420.

67. Luque R, Casilari E, Moron MJ, et al. Comparison and characterization of Android-based fall detection systems. Sensors (Basel) 2014;14(10):18543–74.

68. Rasche P, Mertens A, Brohl C, et al. The "Aachen fall prevention App" - a Smartphone application app for the self-assessment of elderly patients at risk for ground level falls. Patient Saf Surg 2017;11:14.

69. Pape HC, Schemmann U, Foerster J, et al. The 'Aachen Falls Prevention Scale' - development of a tool for self-assessment of elderly patients at risk for ground level falls. Patient Saf Surg 2015;9:7.

70. Gurley RJ, Lum N, Sande M, et al. Persons found in their homes helpless or dead. N Engl J Med 1996;334(26):1710–6.

71. Vilarinho T, Farshchian B, Bajer DG, et al. A combined smartphone and smartwatch fall detection system. Paper presented at: 2015 IEEE International Conference on Computer and Information Technology; Ubiquitous Computing and Communications; Dependable, Autonomic and Secure Computing; Pervasive Intelligence and Computing; Santa Clara (CA), October 26–28, 2015.

72. Patel PA, Gunnarsson C. A passive monitoring system in assisted living facilities: 12-month comparative study. Phys Occup Ther Geriat 2012;30(1):45–52.

The Overlap Between Falls and Delirium in Hospitalized Older Adults: A Systematic Review

Andrea Yevchak Sillner, PhD, GCNS-BC, RN[a,b],
Cynthia L. Holle, DNP, MBA, RN[a], James L. Rudolph, MD, SM[a,c,d],*

KEYWORDS

• Falls • Delirium • Systematic review • Older adults • Hospital

KEY POINTS

• Falls and delirium share many predisposing risk factors and precipitating events.
• Falls are more likely to occur in hospitalized older adults with delirium.
• Patient safety risk screening assessments and interventions, including falls and delirium, should be routinely implemented for all hospitalized individuals older than 65 years.

Older persons are complex. Each individual has a unique milieu of comorbidities, physical limits, psychological experiences, and social supports that affect the ability to respond to stressors. Acute illness stresses the milieu, and some are more vulnerable than others. Adverse events occur in up to 10% of hospitalized persons and add stress to the acute illness.[1,2] Hospitalized older adults are particularly vulnerable to adverse events, which may be related to overall frailty, mobility and balance issues, or frailty-related rates of hospitalization and longer lengths of stay.[3–5] Up to 30% of older adults over the age of 65 years experience a fall, with increasing rates in those older than 80.[6,7] Adverse events for this population may be considered geriatric syndromes, with falls and delirium being particularly common.[8,9] The relationship

Funding: This material is based on work supported by the Office of Academic Affiliations and the Office of Research and Development (R&D), and Health Services R&D (HSR&D) (C.L. Holle). This work was supported by the VA Health Services Research and Development Center of Innovation in Long Term Services and Supports (CIN 13-419) (A.Y. Sillner, C.L. Holle, and J.L. Rudolph) and the VA QUERI-Geriatrics and Extended Care Partnered Evaluation for Community Nursing Homes (PEC 15-465) (J.L. Rudolph).
^a Center of Innovation in Long-Term Services and Supports, Providence VA Medical Center (650), 830 Chalkstone Avenue, Providence, RI 02908 USA; ^b College of Nursing, The Pennsylvania State University, 201 Nursing Sciences Building, University Park, PA 16802, USA; ^c Department of Medicine, Warren Alpert Medical School, Brown University, Box G-A1, Providence, RI 02912, USA; ^d Center of Gerontology and Health Research, Brown University School of Public Health, Providence, RI, USA
* Corresponding author. Department of Medicine, Warren Alpert Medical School, Brown University, Box G-A1, Providence, RI 02912, USA.
E-mail address: james.rudolph@va.gov

between falls and delirium is complex. Falls may contribute to the development of delirium, and delirium may lead to a fall. Therefore, it is important to further understand this relationship.[10,11]

FALLS

In-hospital falls are "never events" according to the Centers for Medicare & Medicaid Services, yet up to 1 million people in the United States experience an in-hospital fall annually. Literature often defines falls as unplanned or sudden events whereby the patient descends to the floor, another person, or other object, with or without injury.[10,11] In older adults, falls, including noninjurious ones, can lead to increased risks of mortality, longer lengths of stay, lowered likelihood of discharge back to the community, decreased ability to perform activities of daily living, and higher costs of care.[10–12] Incident reports are routinely and systematically used to report falls within the hospital, rehabilitation, and nursing homes.[13] Although there are reported inconsistencies in documentation and characterization of falls, these reports are used for patient safety and quality improvement strategies.[14]

DELIRIUM

Delirium is common in hospitalized older adults, with studies suggesting that up to 31% of older adults have delirium on hospital admission and up to 42% will develop incident delirium during hospitalization.[15–17] Delirium is an acute and fluctuating change in attention and cognition, frequently occurring in older adults.[17] In the hospital, delirium remains underdetected and underreported.[18,19] Similar to falls, delirium results in worsened outcomes for hospitalized older adults that persist even after hospital discharge.[20–22]

COMMON RISK FACTORS FOR FALLS AND DELIRIUM IN HOSPITALIZED OLDER ADULTS

Hospitalized older adults experience a complex interaction between individual vulnerabilities and those added by the hospital environment. Within this complex milieu, vulnerability to stress transcends current diagnostic categories. The complexity makes identification of a single, definitive causal link almost impossible. An older adult hospitalized for an acute exacerbation of chronic congestive heart failure, for example, has individual vulnerabilities that can include sarcopenia, presbyopia, and reduced cognitive reserve that typically do not affect function in the usual home environment. When these individual vulnerabilities combine with unique hospital environment features such as medications to induce diuresis, low environmental lighting, and a change in room layout, a fall can easily occur. Determining a single definitive "cause" becomes impossible because of the complex and interdependent milieu.

In the complex milieu, the factors that contribute to one syndrome often contribute to others. "Geriatric syndrome" is a term used to describe conditions that commonly occur in older adults, but do not have a specific diagnosis category[6] and include falls and delirium.[6,7] These syndromes often occur in the most vulnerable older adults, leading to poor outcomes as already described. Syndromes such as falls and delirium have identified personal predisposing factors and precipitating events that increase their likelihood, in the context of the complex interaction of vulnerabilities and stress.

Fall risk factors include arthritis, depression, cognitive impairment, visual disturbances, impaired balance and gait, and the use of 4 or more medications.[12] For older adults there is an even higher risk with a hospitalization, new acute illness, or exacerbation of an existing chronic condition.[12] Prior fall history is also an independent risk factor for subsequent falls and contributes to the "fear of falling" and the lasting psychological impact of falls.[7,23]

Delirium most often occurs in those with preexisting cognitive impairment.[24,25] Additional predisposing factors include increasing age, frailty, lowered functional abilities, and vision and hearing impairment.[25] Hospital precipitating events include acute illness, hospitalization, infection, medications, urinary catheter insertion, electrolyte imbalance, and malnutrition.[25] Malnutrition and dehydration are also considered geriatric syndromes, demonstrating the overlap between these syndromes, risks, and outcomes.[26]

To date there has not been a systematic analysis specific to falls and delirium, despite the significant overlap of falls on delirium and delirium on falls. A recent systematic review and meta-analysis did demonstrate that use of the Hospital Elder Life Program, which is a delirium prevention program, does result in a reduction in falls.[27] The purpose of this article is to examine the underlying literature of delirium and falls and lay a foundation from which future attempts can build an understanding of the complex milieu. In addition, clinicians will have the resource of a practical checklist regarding falls and delirium in hospitalized older adults.

METHODS
Search Method

The study protocol was created a priori according to the Preferred Reporting Items for Systematic Reviews and Meta-Analyses Statement (PRISMA) guidelines and registered with the International Prospective Register of Systematic Reviews (PROSPERO). PROSPERO and the Cochrane Database of Systematic Reviews were searched for related systematic reviews to ensure originality. The search strategy was finalized after independent consultation with a health science librarian.

The search terms are listed in Appendix 1 and included the intersection of falls AND delirium AND hospital care. The search was conducted in the online bibliographic databases PubMed, PsychINFO, CINAHL, and Web of Science from July 18, 2018, with restrictions to English language and age 65 years or older. A copy of the full MeSH and key word search strategy has been provided in an Online Appendix. A search was also completed of the included full-text articles and relevant review reference lists to identify any additional relevant studies. Two authors independently performed data collection, data extraction, and assessment of study quality, with any disagreement resolved by the third author.

Eligibility Criteria

Studies that met the following criteria were included: (1) original or primary peer-reviewed research, observational study design, conducted in adults older than 65 years in any hospital setting, and reported on both delirium and falls as outcomes. Hospital was defined as any inpatient facility that provided primary medical care. Delirium was defined as either prevalent or incident delirium. Studies were excluded for the following: (1) studied a different population (ie, emergency department, long-term care, skilled nursing care, palliative and/or hospice care) or (2) delirium was related to alcohol withdrawal or the presence of alcohol.

Search Outcome

After removal of duplicates, the search strategy yielded a total of 380 records. Two reviewers (AYS and JLR) completed title and abstract screening independently. The

Rayyan Qatar Computing Research Institute Web-based application was used to conduct blind screenings. If either reviewer indicated that a study met inclusion criteria, it was reviewed in full text. A total of 86 full-text articles were assessed for eligibility criteria. Two reviewers completed full-text screenings independently and in duplicate using the standardized eligibility criteria. Disagreements were resolved by discussion or the involvement of a third reviewer. Full-text articles were excluded for the following reasons: (1) they did not report on the interaction of falls and delirium and (2) the outcomes reported did not include both falls and delirium. **Fig. 1** provides a flow diagram of the results of the search and selection process according to PRISMA guidelines.

Study Quality Appraisal

Studies were assessed for risk of bias using the Risk of Bias in Non-Randomized Studies for Interventions (ROBINS-I) tool.[28] However, neither fall nor delirium is ethically inducible, such that a nonbiased randomized study of falls and delirium is

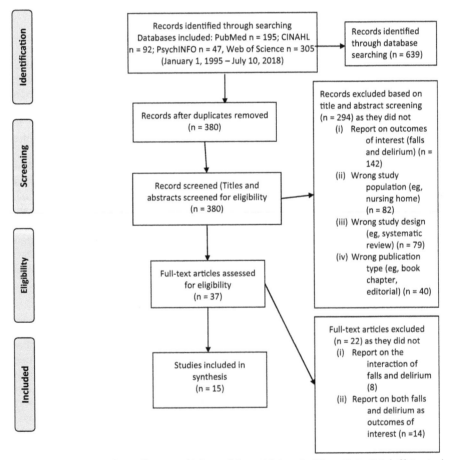

Fig. 1. PRISMA 2009 flow diagram. (*Adapted from* Moher D, Liberati A, Tetzlaff J, et al. Preferred reporting items for systematic reviews and meta-analyses: the PRISMA Statement. PLoS Med 2009;6(7):e1000097.)

impossible (eg, you cannot cause someone to fall or give them delirium). As a result, the intervention elements of the ROBINS-I tool were not included in the bias assessments.

Data Abstraction, Synthesis, and Analysis

Two reviewers' extracted data independently and in duplicate from included studies using a standardized electronic data form developed by the authors. Data elements extracted included study information (eg, author, publication year, study design), patient demographic characteristics (eg, age, sex, education, reason for hospitalization, type of hospital unit, delirium status), delirium assessment, and fall assessment. A third reviewer independently validated abstracted data. The findings were summarized using descriptive statistics including study design and size, characteristics of the population, measurement of the outcomes, and occurrence of the outcomes.

Statistical Methods

Within the analysis cohort for each study, the number of participants was identified with each outcome as well as the number of participants at the intersection of delirium and falls. From this, the risk of the outcome for both delirium and falls was calculated, as well as the risk ratio (RR) for falling with delirium including the 95% confidence interval (CI).

RESULTS

Tables 1 and **2** present the characteristics of the 15 included studies conducted in 7 different countries, primarily the United States (7)[10,29–34] and Australia (3),[35–37] in various types of acute care wards, primarily general medical units[29,31,36–38] or hospital-wide on multiple units.[10,33–35] Most studies reviewed had samples that were primarily female. **Table 1** reports additional characteristics of studies that examined falls in acute care for the presence of delirium. All of these studies used retrospective data-collection methods.[10,33,34,39,40] Methods used for determining the presence of a fall were consistent across the studies; all used incident reports. Delirium diagnosis methods were mixed. Some studies used reliable, validated tools for detection of delirium such as the Confusion Assessment Method (CAM), Confusion Assessment Method Intensive Care Unit (CAM-ICU),[33] or the Intensive Care Delirium Screening Checklist.[40] Others used medical diagnostic codes including the *Diagnostic and Statistical Manual of Mental Disorders, Fourth Edition* or the *International Classification of Diseases, Ninth Revision*.[34] Other studies used expert review[10] as a delirium determination or did not state how the presence of delirium was determined.[39] Sample sizes ranged from 99 to more than 5000. Two of the studies compared cohorts of individuals who fell with those who did not fall.[39,40] Delirium was present in varying degrees in persons who fell, ranging from 24% to 96%.

Table 2 reports characteristics of studies that were examined for the presence of falls and delirium in larger samples. Fall diagnosis methods differed across the studies, with the primary method being medical record review for a fall (4).[29,31,32,41] Three of these studies did not report how they ascertained the diagnosis of a fall,[30,37,42] in contrast to studies reporting on all fallers in **Table 1**, which reported a fall diagnosis method. All studies reported how delirium was diagnosed, with the CAM being the most common tool.[29,32,37,38,42] Sample sizes varied from 97 to more than 3 million. Mean age of study participants was older than 66 years. Fall rates in the samples varied from 1.3% to 100%, whereas delirium occurred from 0.7% to greater than 75% of the participants.

Table 1
Study characteristics of studies that examined falls for the presence of delirium

Authors, Year	Country	Acute Care Ward Type	Study Design	Fall Diagnosis Method	Delirium Diagnosis Method	Sample Size, n	Age, Mean (SD)	Female Gender, n (%)	Individuals with Falls, n (%)	Individuals with Delirium, n (%)
Babine et al,[10] 2016	United States	Multiple	Retrospective, chart review	Incident report	Expert review	99	62.8 (—)	40%	99 (100%)	71 (72%)
Ferguson et al,[33] 2018	United States	Multiple	Retrospective, cohort	Incident report	CAM, CAM-ICU, expert review	7095 patient days/month preintervention	67.5 (16.1)	35 (42%)	2.58/1000 (patient days) ALL FALLS 0.09/1000 (patient days) DELIRIUM FALLS	35.27%
						6596 patient days/month postintervention	68.1 (15.8)	34 (32%)	2.03/1000 (patient days) ALL FALLS 0.05/1000 (patient days) DELIRIUM FALLS	24.63%
Hanger et al,[39] 2014	New Zealand	Rehabilitation	Retrospective, chart review	Incident report	—	122 fallers 279 nonfallers	79.1 79.8	49.2% 55.9%	122 (100%)	58 (24%)
Lakatos et al,[34] 2009	United States	Multiple	Retrospective, chart review	Medical record, incident report	DSM-IV, ICD-9	237	—	48%	237 (100%)	228 (96%)
Trumble et al,[40] 2017	Canada	Intensive care unit	Retrospective, cohort	Medical record	Intensive Care Delirium Screening Checklist	5009 nonfallers 26 fallers	56.3 (17.1) 54.5 (17.4)	1954 (39%) 6 (23%)	0 (0.0%) 26 (100%)	— 13 (50%)

Abbreviations: —, indicates missing data from article review; CAM, confusion assessment method; CAM-ICU, confusion assessment method intensive care unit; DSM-IV, diagnostic and statistical manual of mental disorders, fourth edition; ICD-9, international classification of diseases, ninth revision.

Table 2

Study characteristics of studies that examined for the presence of falls and delirium in a larger sample

Authors, Year	Country	Acute Care Ward Type	Study Design	Fall Diagnosis Method	Delirium Diagnosis Method	Sample Size, n	Age, Mean (SD)	Female Gender, n (%)	Individuals with Falls, n (%)	Individuals with Delirium, n (%)
Basic and Hartwell,[36] 2015	Australia	Medical unit	Prospective cohort	Incident report	Expert review	2945	82.7 (7.6)	1817 (61.7%)	257 (8.7%)	921 (31.3%)
Brand and Sundararajan,[35] 2010	Australia	Multiple	Retrospective, cohort	ICD-10-AM	ICD-10-AM	3,345,415	—	1,952,479 (58.4%)	45,092 (1.3%)	22,077 (0.7%)
Dharmarajan et al,[29] 2017	United States	Medical	Secondary data analysis	Medical record, incident report	CAM, MMSE	469	80.1 (6.5)	282 (60.1%)	14 (3.2%)	70 (14.9%)
Mangusan et al,[30] 2015	United States	Cardiac surgery	Retrospective, chart review	—	Keyword	656	66.5 (10.8)	220 (33.5%)	15 (2.3%)	161 (24.5%)
Mazur et al,[42] 2016	Poland	Geriatric	Prospective, observational	—	CAM	788	79.5 (7.6)	520 (66.0%)	26 (3.3%)	22 (2.8%)

(continued on next page)

Table 2
(continued)

Authors, Year	Country	Acute Care Ward Type	Study Design	Fall Diagnosis Method	Delirium Diagnosis Method	Sample Size, n	Age, Mean (SD)	Female Gender, n (%)	Individuals with Falls, n (%)	Individuals with Delirium, n (%)
Mudge et al,[37] 2013	Australia	Medical	Quality improvement	—	CAM	74 pre 62 post	82.3 (7.7) 79.6 (8.2)	36 (48.6%) 32 (51.6%)	10 (7.4%)	46 (33.8%)
Nanda et al,[32] 2011	United States	Geriatric-psychiatric	Retrospective, chart review	Medical record	CAM	225	79 (7.7)	113 (50%)	136 (64.4%)	151 (67.1%)
Pendlebury et al,[38] 2015	United Kingdom	Medical	Prospective, observational	Observation	CAM	308	81.0 (8.0)	160 (52%)	15 (4.9%)	95 (30.8%)
Stenvall et al,[41] 2006	Sweden	Orthopedic	Prospective	Medical record	MMSE, observation	97	82.0 (5.9)	74 (76%)	26 (26.8%)	73 (75.3%)
Wakefield,[31] 2002	United States	Medical	Prospective, cohort	Medical record	NEECHAM	117	73 (4.6)	117 (100%)	6 (5.1%)	16 (13.7%)

Abbreviations: —, indicates missing data from article review; CAM, confusion assessment method; ICD-10-AM, *international classification of diseases, tenth revision, Australian modification*; MMSE, mini-mental state examination; NEECHAM, Neelon and Champagne Confusion Scale.

Table 3 details the numbers of fallers, nonfallers, and risk of incident falls (per patient) for those with and without delirium. The median risk of falling with delirium among the studies was 12% (range from 6% to 67%) with smaller studies on the higher end of the range. The risk of falling was lower among the comparison group without delirium in all studies (median 2%, range 1% to 47%). Accordingly, the RR for falls with delirium was elevated and significant in all studies but one (median RR = 4.5, range 1.4–12.6). **Fig. 2** displays this graphically in a forest plot. A pooled RR was not calculated because of the heterogeneity of the studies, risk for bias, and limitations of the studies.

DISCUSSION

In this systematic review, 5 studies that assessed delirium among fallers and 10 studies that measured delirium, falls, and the interaction were identified. In general, delirium is more common among fallers and there is a consistently elevated risk of falls among patients with delirium. Although there are limitations and biases that limit a pooled analysis, clinicians can recognize the inextricable association of delirium and falls, and a combined patient safety approach may be necessary to mitigate negative consequences of either.

Delirium and falls may share a common cognitive deficit. The hallmark cognitive deficit of delirium is impaired inattention. Attention is the cognitive process of selectively concentrating on one aspect of the environment while ignoring other things.[43] Although falls occur for numerous reasons, most falls occur at night among patients who are trying to go to the bathroom.[44] Impaired attention, such as that in delirium, limits the recognition and interpretation of multiple environmental stimuli in the hospital, which might serve as a warning flag to the hospitalized patient that they are at risk for falls. Examples of these warning flags can include urinary catheters, reduced strength and stability, poor environmental lighting, or simply not being able to locate the bathroom. In addition, a separate meta-analysis found that the common cognitive deficit might suggest that preventing delirium prevents falls.[27]

Studies in delirium have found that delirium is underrecognized across staff including physicians, nurses, and nursing assistants, particularly in persons with pre-existing dementia.[19] This systematic underidentification is likely multifactorial with causes including a knowledge deficit, lack of clinically useful delirium assessment tools, and, most importantly, inattention to the time constraints of modern nursing.[18,19] Development and validation of a patient safety risk algorithm, embedded in the electronic medical record (EMR), which encompasses falls and delirium, may provide efficient clinical utility for risk identification by acute care providers.

Despite the high risk of falls in patients with delirium, the common fall risk tools are inconsistent with delirium terminology. **Table 4** includes the terminology for cognitive impairment in common falls scales. Although instructions accompanying the forms often include specific terms such as impulsivity, disorientation, and inability to follow commands, these terms are relatively nonspecific and do not include an objective assessment of cognitive function. For delirium, the 1987 release of the *Diagnostic and Statistical Manual of Mental Disorders, Third Edition—Revised* was an important innovation that defined the syndrome and clarified the central role of inattention.[45] In subsequent years, this led to systematic algorithms to diagnose delirium and, more recently, operationalized tools for assessment.[46,47] Given the advancements in cognitive assessment and a stronger understanding of the association of delirium and falls, consideration should be provided to stronger inclusion of delirium and likely reweighting of falls algorithms. Even more important, the ubiquity of EMRs, including historical diagnosis and utilization data elements and the emerging machine learning

Table 3
Relative risk ratios for studies that identified the interaction of falls and delirium

Authors, Year	Risk of Bias	Total, n	Delirium			No Delirium			Risk for Fall with Delirium
			Fall, n	No Fall, n	Risk, %	Fall, n	No Fall, n	Risk, %	RR (95% CI)
Basic and Hartwell,[36] 2015	Serious	2945	131	790	14.2	126	1898	6.2	2.28 (1.81, 2.88)
Brand and Sundararajan,[35] 2010	Serious	3,345,415	1325	20,752	6.0	43,767	3,279,571	1.3	4.56 (4.32, 4.81)
Dharmarajan et al,[29] 2017	Moderate	469	6	64	8.5	8	391	2.0	4.23 (1.53, 11.95)
Mangusan et al,[30] 2015	Serious	656	10	151	6.2	5	490	1.0	6.14 (2.13, 17.73)
Mazur et al,[42] 2016	Moderate	788	2	20	9.1	24	742	3.1	2.90 (0.73, 11.52)
Mudge et al,[37] 2011	Serious	136	8	38	17.4	2	88	2.2	7.83 (1.73, 35.36)
Nanda et al,[32] 2011	Serious	225	101	50	66.9	35	39	47.3	1.41 (1.08, 1.84)
Pendlebury et al,[38] 2015	Moderate	308	10	85	10.5	5	208	2.3	4.48 (1.58, 12.76)
Stenvall et al,[41] 2006	Moderate	97	25	48	34.2	1	23	4.2	8.22 (1.18, 57.47)
Wakefield,[31] 2002	Serious	117	4	12	25.0	2	99	2.0	12.63 (2.51, 63.37)

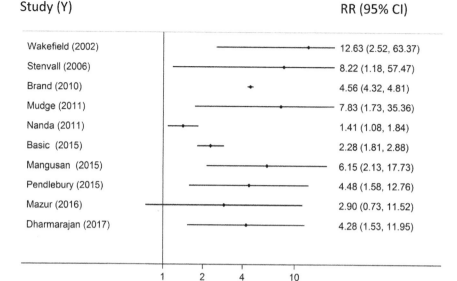

Fig. 2. Forest plot of studies that identified the interaction of delirium and falls. The forest plot demonstrates the risk ratio for falls with and without delirium. CI, confidence interval; RR, risk ratio.

field, offer an opportunity to streamline risk assessment instruments[48] for delirium, falls, and patient safety simultaneously.

We propose a streamlined patient safety algorithm (**Fig. 3**) including fall and delirium risk assessments and intervention sets. This type of model can be modified according to the unique setting, and can also include additional factors as they become known. This type of approach can be used to structure communication during transitions of care so that risk factors are known and documented consistently.

Table 4
Terms used for cognitive impairment in fall risk assessment scales

Scale Name	Cognitive Impairment Term (Points)	Additional Cognitive Impairment Description if Provided in Scale (Points)	Total Points (High-Risk Cutoff)
Morse Fall Scale	Mental status (15)	• Knows own limits (0) • Overestimates or forgets limits (15)	125 (46+)
Hendrich II Fall Risk Model	Confusion/ disorientation/ impulsivity (4)	N/A	20 (5)
STRATIFY Scale for Identifying Fall Risk Factors	Agitated (1)	Is the patient agitated? (1)	5 (2)
John Hopkins Fall Risk Assessment Tool	Cognition (7)	• Altered awareness of immediate physical environment (1) • Impulsive (2) • Lack of understanding of one's physical and cognitive limitations (4)	35 (13)

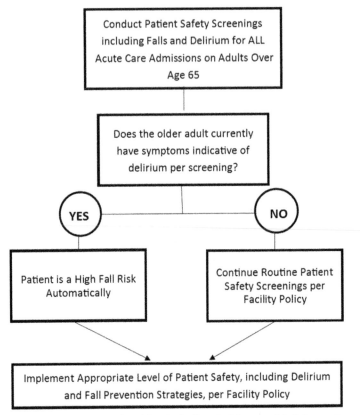

Fig. 3. Patient Safety Screening Algorithm including Delirium and Fall Prevention.

This systematic review has several notable strengths and limitations. Strengths include the development of an inclusive and extensive hypothesis-driven systematic review search strategy in consultation with a health sciences librarian. There was independent expert review of the articles and a bias assessment conducted of the included studies. The weakness of this systematic review is that it included observational, retrospective, and chart review studies, some with biases that limited meta-analysis. However, there was a consistent association between falls and delirium. An additional limitation is that 2 of the articles had samples that included individuals across the 65-year-old cutoff, and these included age cutoff data for falls and delirium.[35,40]

SUMMARY

This systematic review found that delirium is more common among fallers, and there is a consistently elevated risk of falls among patients with delirium. Falls and delirium share many risk factors and should be considered within a common patient safety pathway for routine assessment, prevention, and management in hospitalized older adults.

ACKNOWLEDGMENTS

Drs A.Y. Sillner, C.L. Holle and J.L. Rudolph are employees of the United States Department of Veterans Affairs (VA). The opinions expressed here are those of the authors and do not represent the policies and positions of the VA.

REFERENCES

1. de Vries EN, Ramrattan MA, Smorenburg SM, et al. The incidence and nature of in-hospital adverse events: a systematic review. Qual Saf Health Care 2008;17(3): 216–23.
2. Zegers M, Hesselink G, Geense W, et al. Evidence-based interventions to reduce adverse events in hospitals: a systematic review of systematic reviews. BMJ Open 2016;6(9):e012555.
3. Tsilimingras D, Rosen AK, Berlowitz DR. Patient safety in geriatrics: a call for action. J Gerontol A Biol Sci Med Sci 2003;58(9):M813–9.
4. Theou O, Squires E, Mallery K, et al. What do we know about frailty in the acute care setting? A scoping review. BMC Geriatr 2018;18(1):139.
5. Juma S, Taabazuing M-M, Montero-Odasso M. Clinical frailty scale in an acute medicine unit: a simple tool that predicts length of stay. Can Geriatr J 2016; 19(2):34–9.
6. Inouye SK, Studenski S, Tinetti ME, et al. Geriatric syndromes: clinical, research and policy implications of a core geriatric concept. J Am Geriatr Soc 2007;55(5): 780–91.
7. Tinetti ME, Kumar C. The patient who falls: "it's always a trade-off". JAMA 2010; 303(3):258–66.
8. Morley JE. Rapid geriatric assessment. Clin Geriatr Med 2017;33(3):431–40.
9. Lee EA, Gibbs NE, Fahey L, et al. Making hospitals safer for older adults: updating quality metrics by understanding hospital-acquired delirium and its link to falls. Perm J 2013;17(4):32–6.
10. Babine RL, Hyrkäs KE, Bachand DA, et al. Falls in a tertiary care hospital—association with delirium: a replication study. Psychosomatics 2016;57(3):273–82.
11. Babine RL, Hyrkäs KE, Hallen S, et al. Falls and delirium in an acute care setting: a retrospective chart review before and after an organisation-wide interprofessional education. J Clin Nurs 2018;27(7/8):e1429–41.
12. Tinetti ME. Preventing falls in elderly persons. N Engl J Med 2003;348(1):42–9.
13. Toyabe S. Characteristics of inpatient falls not reported in an incident reporting system. Glob J Health Sci 2016;8(3):17–25.
14. Simon M, Klaus S, Gajewski BJ, et al. Agreement of fall classifications among staff in U.S. hospitals. Nurs Res 2013;62(2):74–81.
15. Ryan DJ, O'Regan NA, Caoimh RÓ, et al. Delirium in an adult acute hospital population: predictors, prevalence and detection. BMJ Open 2013;3(1) [pii: e001772].
16. Bellelli G, Morandi A, Di Santo SG, et al. "Delirium Day": a nationwide point prevalence study of delirium in older hospitalized patients using an easy standardized diagnostic tool. BMC Med 2016;14:106.
17. Siddiqi N, House AO, Holmes JD. Occurrence and outcome of delirium in medical in-patients: a systematic literature review. Age Ageing 2006;35(4):350–64.
18. Steis MR, Behrens L, Colancecco EM, et al. Licensed nurse and nursing assistant recognition of delirium in nursing home residents with dementia. Ann Longterm Care 2015;23(10):15–20.
19. Steis MR, Fick DM. Delirium superimposed on dementia: accuracy of nurse documentation. J Gerontol Nurs 2012;38(1):32–42.
20. Cole M, McCusker J, Dendukuri N, et al. The prognostic significance of subsyndromal delirium in elderly medical inpatients. J Am Geriatr Soc 2003;51(6): 754–60.

21. Fick DM, Steis MR, Waller JL, et al. Delirium superimposed on dementia is associated with prolonged length of stay and poor outcomes in hospitalized older adults. J Hosp Med 2013;8(9):500–5.
22. Khan BA, Zawahiri M, Campbell NL, et al. Delirium in hospitalized patients: implications of current evidence on clinical practice and future avenues for research–a systematic evidence review. J Hosp Med 2012;7(7):580–9.
23. Boltz M, Resnick B, Capezuti E, et al. Activity restriction vs. self-direction: hospitalised older adults' response to fear of falling. Int J Older People Nurs 2014;9(1):44–53.
24. Fong TG, Davis D, Growdon ME, et al. The interface between delirium and dementia in elderly adults. Lancet Neurol 2015;14(8):823–32.
25. Ahmed S, Leurent B, Sampson EL. Risk factors for incident delirium among older people in acute hospital medical units: a systematic review and meta-analysis. Age Ageing 2014;43(3):326–33.
26. Anderson CP, Ngo LH, Marcantonio ER. Complications in postacute care are associated with persistent delirium. J Am Geriatr Soc 2012;60(6):1122–7.
27. Hshieh TT, Yang T, Gartaganis SL, et al. Hospital elder life program: systematic review and meta-analysis of effectiveness. Am J Geriatr Psychiatry 2018;26(10):1015–33.
28. Sterne JA, Hernán MA, Reeves BC, et al. ROBINS-I: a tool for assessing risk of bias in non-randomised studies of interventions. BMJ 2016;355:i4919.
29. Dharmarajan K, Swami S, Gou RY, et al. Pathway from delirium to death: potential in-hospital mediators of excess mortality. J Am Geriatr Soc 2017;65(5):1026–33.
30. Mangusan RF, Hooper V, Denslow SA, et al. Outcomes associated with postoperative delirium after cardiac surgery. Am J Crit Care 2015;24(2):156–63.
31. Wakefield BJ. Behaviors and outcomes of acute confusion in hospitalized patients. Appl Nurs Res 2002;15(4):209–16.
32. Nanda S, Dey T, Gulstrand RE Jr, et al. Fall risk assessment in geriatric-psychiatric inpatients to lower events (FRAGILE). J Gerontol Nurs 2011;37(2):22–30 [quiz: 32–23].
33. Ferguson A, Uldall K, Dunn J, et al. Effectiveness of a multifaceted delirium screening, prevention, and treatment initiative on the rate of delirium falls in the acute care setting. J Nurs Care Qual 2018;33(3):213–20.
34. Lakatos BE, Capasso V, Mitchell MT, et al. Falls in the general hospital: association with delirium, advanced age, and specific surgical procedures. Psychosomatics 2009;50(3):218–26.
35. Brand CA, Sundararajan V. A 10-year cohort study of the burden and risk of in-hospital falls and fractures using routinely collected hospital data. Qual Saf Health Care 2010;19(6):e51.
36. Basic D, Hartwell TJ. Falls in hospital and new placement in a nursing home among older people hospitalized with acute illness. Clin Interv Aging 2015;10:1637–43.
37. Mudge AM, Maussen C, Duncan J, et al. Improving quality of delirium care in a general medical service with established interdisciplinary care: a controlled trial. Intern Med J 2013;43(3):270–7.
38. Pendlebury S, Lovett N, Smith S, et al. Observational, longitudinal study of delirium in consecutive unselected acute medical admissions: age-specific rates and associated factors, mortality and re-admission. BMJ Open 2015;5(11):e007808.
39. Hanger HC, Wills KL, Wilkinson T. Classification of falls in stroke rehabilitation—not all falls are the same. Clin Rehabil 2014;28(2):183–95.

40. Trumble D, Meier MA, Doody M, et al. Incidence, correlates and outcomes associated with falls in the intensive care unit: a retrospective cohort study. Crit Care Resusc 2017;19(4):290–5.

41. Stenvall M, Olofsson B, Lundström M, et al. Inpatient falls and injuries in older patients treated for femoral neck fracture. Arch Gerontol Geriatr 2006;43(3):389–99.

42. Mazur K, Wilczyński K, Szewieczek J. Geriatric falls in the context of a hospital fall prevention program: delirium, low body mass index, and other risk factors. Clin Interv Aging 2016;11:1253–61.

43. Anderson D. Preventing delirium in older people. Br Med Bull 2005;73-74:25–34.

44. Hitcho EB, Krauss MJ, Birge S, et al. Characteristics and circumstances of falls in a hospital setting: a prospective analysis. J Gen Intern Med 2004;19(7):732–9.

45. American Psychiatric Association: Diagnostic and Statistical Manual of Mental Disorders, 3rd edition, revised. Washington, DC: American Psychiatric Association, 1987.

46. Bellelli G, Morandi A, Davis DHJ, et al. Validation of the 4AT, a new instrument for rapid delirium screening: a study in 234 hospitalised older people. Age Ageing 2014;43(4):496–502.

47. Ely E, Shintani A, Truman B, et al. Delirium as a predictor of mortality in mechanically ventilated patients in the intensive care unit. JAMA 2004;291(14):1753–62.

48. Rudolph JL, Doherty K, Kelly B, et al. Validation of a delirium risk assessment using electronic medical record information. J Am Med Dir Assoc 2016;17(3):244–8.

APPENDIX 1: MeSH AND KEYWORD SEARCH STRATEGIES FOR EACH DATABASE

Web of Science Search Total 305 (search ran on 7/10/18)
Search Limits: English Language
("accidental falls" OR "falls" OR "falling" OR "slip and fall" OR "accidental fall" OR "fall") AND ("delirium" OR "acute psychosis" OR "acute psychoses" OR "psychosis" OR "psychoses" OR "icu syndrome" OR "ICU psychosis" OR "ICU psychoses" OR "acute confusional state" OR "acute confusional syndrome" OR "acute brain dysfunction") AND ("hospitals" OR "hospital" OR "acute care" OR "inpatients" OR "hospitalized patients" OR "hospitalized patient" OR "inpatient" OR "intensive care units" OR "critical care unit" OR "critical care units" OR "intensive care unit" OR "CCU" OR "ICU" OR "health facilities")
PsychINFO Search TOTAL 47 (search ran on 7/10/18)
Search Limits: English Language; Aged 65 years +
((MAINSUBJECT.EXACT("Falls") OR ab(("accidental falls" OR "accidental fall" OR falls OR fall OR falling OR "slip and fall")) OR ti(("accidental falls" OR "accidental fall" OR falls OR fall OR falling OR "slip and fall"))) AND (MAINSUBJECT.EXACT("Delirium") OR ab((delirium OR "icu Psychosis" OR" icu psychoses" OR "acute brain dysfunction" OR "acute psychosis" OR "acute psychoses" OR psychosis OR psychoses OR "icu syndrome" OR "acute confusional syndrome" OR "acute confusional state")) OR ti((delirium OR "icu Psychosis" OR" icu psychoses" OR "acute brain dysfunction" OR "acute psychosis" OR "acute psychoses" OR psychosis OR psychoses OR "icu syndrome" OR "acute confusional syndrome" OR "acute confusional state"))) AND ((MAINSUBJECT.EXACT("Hospitals") OR MAINSUBJECT.EXACT("Hospitalized Patients")) OR ab(("acute care" OR inpatient OR inpatients OR "hospitalized patients" OR "hospitalized patient" OR "icu" OR "ccu" OR "intensive care unit" OR "intensive care units" OR "critical care unit" OR "critical care units" OR "health facilities" OR hospital OR hospitals)) OR ti(("acute care" OR inpatient OR inpatients

OR "icu" OR "ccu" OR "intensive care unit" OR "intensive care units" OR "critical care unit" OR "critical care units" OR "health facilities" OR hospital OR hospitals))))

CINAHL Search TOTAL 92 (search ran on 7/10/18)

Search Limits: English Language; Aged 65 years +

(((MH "Accidental Falls") OR TI ("accidental falls" OR "accidental fall" OR falls OR fall OR falling OR "slip and fall") OR AB ("accidental falls" OR "accidental fall" OR falls OR fall OR falling OR "slip and fall")) AND

(((MH "Delirium") OR (MH "ICU Psychosis")) OR TI (delirium OR "ICU Psychosis" OR "icu psychoses" OR "acute brain dysfunction" OR "acute psychosis" OR "acute psychoses" OR psychosis OR psychoses OR "ICU syndrome" OR "acute confusional syndrome" OR "acute confusional state") OR AB (delirium OR "ICU Psychosis" OR "acute brain dysfunction" OR "acute psychosis" OR "acute psychoses" OR psychosis OR psychoses OR "ICU syndrome" OR "acute confusional syndrome" OR "acute confusional state")) AND ((MH "Health Facilities") OR TI ("acute care" OR inpatient OR inpatients OR "hospitalized patients" OR "hospitalized patient" OR "ICU" OR "CCU" OR "intensive care unit" OR "intensive care units" OR "critical care unit" OR "critical care units" OR hospital or hospitals) OR AB ("acute care" OR inpatient OR inpatients OR "ICU" OR "CCU" OR "intensive care unit" OR "intensive care units" OR "critical care unit" OR "critical care units" OR hospital or hospitals)))

PubMed Search TOTAL 195 (search ran on 7/10/18)

Search Limits: English Language; Aged 65 years +

("accidental falls"[MeSH Terms] OR "falls"[TIA47, B] OR "falling"[TIAB] OR "slip and fall" [TIAB] OR "accidental falls"[TIAB] OR "accidental fall" [TIAB] OR "fall"[TIAB]) AND ("delirium"[MeSH Terms] OR "delirium" [TIAB] OR "acute psychosis" [TIAB] OR "acute psychoses" [TIAB] OR "psychosis" [TIAB] OR "psychoses" [TIAB] OR "icu syndrome"[TIAB] OR "ICU psychosis" [TIAB] OR "ICU psychoses" [TIAB] OR "acute confusional state" [TIAB] OR "acute confusional syndrome" [TIAB] OR "acute brain dysfunction" [TIAB]) AND ("hospitals"[MeSH Terms] OR "hospitals"[TIAB] OR "hospital"[TIAB] OR "acute care"[TIAB] OR "inpatients"[MeSH Terms] OR "inpatients"[TIAB] OR "inpatient"[TIAB] OR "hospitalized patients" [TIAB] OR "hospitalized patient" [TIAB] OR "intensive care units"[MeSH Terms] OR "intensive care units"[TIAB] OR "critical care unit"[TIAB] OR "critical care units"[TIAB] OR "intensive care unit"[TIAB] OR "CCU"[TIAB] OR "ICU"[TIAB]) AND (English[lang] AND "aged"[MeSH Terms])

Optimizing Function and Physical Activity in Hospitalized Older Adults to Prevent Functional Decline and Falls

Barbara Resnick, PhD, CRNP[a],*, Marie Boltz, PhD, CRNP[b]

KEYWORDS

- Optimizing function • Optimizing physical activity • Hospitalized older adults
- Functional decline • Falls

KEY POINTS

- Physical activity, defined as bodily movement that expends energy, including such things as bed mobility, transfers, bathing, dressing, and walking, has a positive impact on physical and psychosocial outcomes among older adults during their hospitalization and the post hospitalization recovery period.
- The benefits of physical activity continue post hospitalization, with ongoing improvement in function, physical activity, resilience, quality of life, and decreased rates of rehospitalization.
- There is no evidence, however, to recommend a specific type or amount of physical activity needed to achieve beneficial outcomes. It is likely that this varies based on the needs of the patient and the type of acute event that he or she has experienced.

INTRODUCTION

Physical activity, defined as bodily movement that expends energy, including such things as bed mobility, transfers, bathing, dressing, and walking, has a positive impact on physical and psychosocial outcomes among older adults during their hospitalization and the post hospitalization recovery period. A review of 36 studies[1,2] concluded that physical activity during hospitalization resulted in less pain,[3–5] less delirium,[6,7] improved cognition,[8–10] and quality of life,[8–10] and fewer deep vein thromboses,[11,12]

Disclosure: The authors have nothing to disclose.
[a] University of Maryland School of Nursing, 655 West Lombard Street, Baltimore, MD 21201, USA; [b] Pennsylvania State University, College of Nursing, 201 Nursing Sciences Building, University Park, PA 16802, USA
* Corresponding author.
E-mail address: resnick@umaryland.edu

Clin Geriatr Med 35 (2019) 237–251
https://doi.org/10.1016/j.cger.2019.01.003
0749-0690/19/© 2019 Elsevier Inc. All rights reserved.

urinary tract infections,[13,14] and incidences of pneumonia.[7,13,15] In addition, there was no evidence that physical activity during hospitalization increased falls[15,16] or other adverse events,[8,14,17–24] and it decreased readmissions following discharge.[10,25,26] The benefits of physical activity continue post hospitalization, with ongoing improvement in function, physical activity, resilience, quality of life, and decreased rates of re-hospitalization.[10,25,26] There is no evidence, however, to recommend a specific type or amount of physical activity needed to achieve beneficial outcomes. It is likely that this varies based on the needs of the patient and the type of acute event that he or she has experienced.

CHALLENGES TO INCREASING PHYSICAL ACTIVITY AMONG HOSPITALIZED OLDER ADULTS

Despite the known benefits, physical activity is not routinely encouraged and older hospitalized medical patients engage in very low levels of activity,[5,16,27–35] spending at least 80% of their acute care stay in bed.[27] There are patient factors, environment and policy issues, and medical and nursing interventions that limit physical activity.[27,32,36–41] Patient factors include age, sociodemographic characteristics, preexisting disability and disease states, delirium, cognitive status, anemia, pain, fear of falling or exacerbating underlying illnesses, depression, motivation, nutritional status, obesity, sedation, and polypharmacy. Obesity, or the increase in fat mass, is a major contributor to physical function and activity in older adults.[42,43] The coexistence of sarcopenia and obesity (also referred to as sarcopenic obesity) further exacerbates function and activity.[42,43] Additional contributing factors include the attitudes and beliefs of patients, families, and providers, such as the belief that rest facilitates recovery and fear that activity will exacerbate disease or cause falls.[9,44–48]

Acute care environments generally provide limited opportunity for physical activity. The bed is often the only furniture in the hospital room, and the height of the bed or chairs may limit the patient's ability to transfer. Even when patients are encouraged to get out of bed, there generally are no pleasant walking areas or destinations, and patients are restricted from walking to tests and procedures.[2] Policies tend to focus on fall prevention and infection control rather than encouraging physical activity and preventing functional decline.[2,5,25] Best practice recommendations such as Awakening and Breathing Coordination, Delirium monitoring/management, and Early exercise/mobility have not been integrated into the operations of medical and surgical units, confined only to patients who are in intensive care units on ventilatory support, and are geared mainly around decreasing delirium.[49] There are no policies that require reporting of medical patients' physical activity during hospitalization, and no requirements to include physical activity as part of the discharge plan. Finally, even though functional status is considered a critical geriatric "vital sign," unlike falls or catheter-associated urinary tract infections, it is not monitored as a quality measure in acute care.

Medical and nursing interventions that limit physical activity and contribute to functional decline include the tethering effects of indwelling urinary catheters, sequential compression devices, pulse oximetry, wall oxygen, and lack of easily accessible portable oxygen, cardiac monitoring, as well as sedating medications, insufficient or excessive management of pain, and limited food/fluid intake.[20,32,50,51]

Despite the benefits, physical activity is not a focus of care provided in the acute care setting.[9,44,52] In addition, older hospitalized patients themselves do not expect to be physically active during their hospital stay.[53] Physicians and other clinicians in acute care focus on the assessment and management of the acute presenting illness to the exclusion of promoting functional maintenance or recovery. Consequently, there is a lack of focus on the patient's underlying physical capability and function before admission.[47,48,54–56] Nurses in acute care focus on ongoing physical assessments, medication administration, indirect care activities,[2,5,57,58] and, in some situations, provide inappropriate adherence to tethering (eg, use of unnecessary pulse oximetry and/or vital sign monitoring). Conversely, little time is spent by nurses encouraging physical activity.[2,5,34,50,52,59,60] In addition, nurses do not routinely evaluate patients' function and physical capability, and tend to limit self-care by performing functional tasks for patients. This further limits opportunities for physical activity on the part of patients.[34,35,37,50,61,62] Therapy, when ordered and initiated, is often limited to an evaluation before discharge to determine the level of care needed.[63]

FALLS AND FEAR OF FALLING

Falls and a subsequent fear of falling among patients, families, and health care providers have a negative impact on physical activity[16,64,65] as there continues to be a belief among many that limiting activity will reduce the risk of falls.[66] Falls are common among older hospitalized patients, occurring at a rate of 3.56 falls per 1000 patient days.[67] Of these, 25% to 50% result in an injury[68,69] and account for 40% of all adverse events in hospitals.[68] In addition to the physical impact of a fall such as a fracture, skin tear, or head trauma, falls can result in anxiety, fear of falling, loss of self-efficacy associated with performance of activities of daily living, particularly ambulation and social isolation, and lead to longer lengths of stay and increased functional decline. Older hospitalized patients have reported that they were unaware of their individual fall risk factors and what specific activities they should do to decrease the risk.[66] Older patients, however, are willing to engage in fall prevention activities and to be partners with members of the health care team in preventing falls.[66] The presence of cognitive impairment, which is noted in at least 25% of hospitalized older adults,[70,71] challenges engagement. Older adults with cognitive impairment are 2 to 4 times as likely to fall during a hospitalization than those who are not impaired.[72] Providing fall prevention recommendations as is commonly done via signs such as "Call Don't Fall" and "encourage the use of call light" are not likely to be effective for these high-risk individuals as they are unable to retain the falls prevention education and recommendations provided.[73]

Risk factors for falls are both intrinsic to the individual as well as extrinsic and include: limited physical function, impaired vision, impaired cognition and mood, and physical illness, such as orthostatic hypotension, medication side effects, and environmental hazards.[74–76] For older adults with cognitive impairment, the risk factors also include the type and severity of the dementia, behavioral symptoms such as wandering, psychological factors including agitation and depression, psychotropic medication use, restraints, and disease-specific changes that alter gait and balance and a prior history of falls.[74–77] Most falls in acute care settings seem to occur during toileting and when patients, particularly those with cognitive impairment, are left unsupervised in their rooms.[78,79]

INNOVATIVE APPROACHES TO INCREASE PHYSICAL ACTIVITY AND DECREASE FALLS

Although there have been numerous interventions and approaches attempted to increase physical activity among hospitalized older adults and decrease falls, there is no single approach that is noted to be effective.[80,81] Individualized multifactorial interventions, which are interventions that focus on decreasing the specific risk factors for falls for each older patient, are noted to be the most effective fall prevention approaches in community-based settings.[82] Multifactorial interventions for fall prevention include approaches such as physical activity, particularly strength and balance exercises, environmental modification, medication reviews, and modification of individual risk factors (eg, vision loss and incontinence).

THE USE OF VISUAL MEMORY INTERVENTIONS TO PREVENT FALLS

Building off the finding that most falls occur among those with cognitive impairment and during toileting activities, a group in Australia[79] developed a visual memory intervention to decrease fall rates among hospitalized older adults. The visual memory intervention involved exposing older patients to a silent 3-minute video that the group developed, which used universal body language to teach patients to ask for help when they want to ambulate to the toilet. The correct model of asking for help to go to the bathroom is demonstrated, as is the wrong method of trying to go to the bathroom alone and falling. The silent video has the advantage of overcoming language barriers and of engaging older adults with cognitive impairment because it draws on emotional memory and how it feels to fall.

Pilot, feasibility testing of the visual memory intervention did not demonstrate significant improvements in function, physical activity, or a decrease in falls. Recommendations from this study included co-locating older adults when hospitalized, particularly those with cognitive impairment and those with a high risk of falls, and using the video with this high-risk group. Co-locating patients to a single room that is easily visualized by nurses resulted in a decrease in falls, such that there was only 1 fall among 39 patients (2 per 1000 patient bed days) versus 39 falls in the single rooms (5 per 1000 patient bed days).

BED ALARMS AND OTHER TECHNOLOGY INTERVENTIONS

There has not been strong evidence for the effectiveness for bed alarms in terms of prevention of falls or injuries related to falls.[80,83–85] Nurses have reported that bed alarms are useful in alerting them that a patient has got up, but hourly evaluations and monitoring are needed to help prevent the patient for getting up alone. One pilot study[86] that used a bed-exit alarm based on a body-worn accelerometer was noted to decrease the number of falls. However, ongoing work is needed to confirm the findings and address the cost of the intervention and ease of use of the device.

In-room webcams have also been tested as a way in which to prevent inpatient falls.[87] The use of the webcams resulted in a decrease in fall rate per 1000 admissions, but there was no difference in fall rate per 1000 patient days. Ongoing research is needed, particularly with regard to patient acceptance of this type of intervention. The use of wireless technology has also been used to improve nurse communication and thereby facilitate response time among nurses when a patient gets out of bed or engages in an activity that increases the risk of a fall.[88] This approach, as noted, has advantages in terms of early alerting of staff, but it did not result in a decrease in falls.

SYSTEM AND ENVIRONMENTAL INTERVENTIONS

System- and environment-based interventions also have been implemented to prevent falls. The system-based intervention[89] incorporated 4 approaches: (1) wake em, take em; (2) timed toileting, which included toileting the patient 3 times per 8-hour shift; (3) assist in and out of bed; and (4) shoulder safety by helping with all transfers in the first 24 hours post shoulder surgery. All of these approaches focused on supervising older patients when getting out of bed and engaging patients in frequent toileting. This approach resulted in a significant decrease in falls and in falls with injury.[89] Environment approaches to falls prevention when used alone were not as effective.

Another innovative approach to fall prevention, referred to as the Fall Prevention Room,[90] was pilot tested among a group of 11 older adults. The Fall Prevention Room included various fall prevention devices: low beds, shower mats, non-skid double sided socks and slippers, floor cushions, hipsters, and bed alarms. Pilot testing of this intervention resulted in 4 falls over the study period, 3 in the control group and 1 in the treatment group. There was not a statistically significant difference noted between the groups. Replication research is needed to adequately establish the effectiveness of this intervention.

An environment-focused intervention, referred to as the 6-PACK falls prevention program,[84] has also been pilot tested. The 6-PACK program included a fall risk assessment, "falls alert" signs, supervision with toileting, placing walking aids within patient reach, toileting regimes, low-low beds (adjustable height low beds that can be lowered to 2 inches from the floor) and bed/chair alarms. Feasibility testing of this approach was done and the nurses supported the use of the fall risk assessment, the use of low-low beds, and alert signs, but did not find that keeping walking devices within reach was helpful. Further they expressed some concerns about the practicality of low-low beds and helping patients with toileting due to lack of sufficient staff. Effectiveness of the 6-PACK approach has yet to be tested.

INTERVENTIONS TO INCREASE PHYSICAL ACTIVITY

Increasing physical activity among hospitalized older adults is likewise best addressed by taking a multifactorial approach that incorporates a behavior change methodology using the Social Ecological Model[91,92] and Social Cognitive Theory.[93] The Social Ecological Model includes a focus on intrapersonal factors, interpersonal factors to facilitate motivation, environmental issues and policy. Social Cognitive Theory guides the interpersonal interactions between patients, families, nurses and other health care team members that can motivate patients to engage in physical activity. Social Cognitive Theory includes self-efficacy, defined as the belief that one can organize and execute a course of action to achieve a specific goal and outcome expectations, which are the beliefs that if a certain behavior is performed it will lead to an anticipated outcome. The stronger the individual's self-efficacy and outcome expectations the more likely it is that he or she will initiate and persist with an activity. Efficacy expectations are enhanced by 4 mechanisms[93-95]: (1) enactive mastery experience; (2) verbal encouragement; (3) vicarious experience; and (4) affective states such as anxiety associated with an activity.

FUNCTION-FOCUSED CARE FOR ACUTE CARE

The Function Focused Care for Acute Care (FFC-AC) intervention is one approach that has been used to increase physical activity among older hospitalized patients and prevent functional decline, falls, and other adverse events such as infections and delirium.[5,26,60,96-98] Function-focused care is a philosophy of care that teaches health care providers and lay caregivers to evaluate older adults' underlying capability with regard to function and physical activity and optimize the older individual's participation in all activities. The advantage of function-focused care is that it can be implemented on diverse hospital units and integrated into the daily operations of the unit. Function-focused care activities are practical and individualized and include engaging patients in bed mobility, bathing, dressing, and ambulating. Examples of function-focused care interactions include: modeling functional behavior for patients (eg, oral care, eating); providing verbal cues during activities of daily living such as dressing; walking a resident to the bathroom or for radiography rather than transporting via wheelchair; doing resistance and balance exercises with patients; and providing recreational physical activity (eg, Physical Activity Bingo). Implementation of FFC-AC includes 4 steps: (1) environment and policy assessments; (2) education of staff on function-focused care; (3) establishing patient goals; and (4) ongoing mentoring and motivating of staff, patients, and families (**Table 1**). In efficacy trials, FFC-AC altered hospital environments and policies to facilitate physical activity,[5,96,99] increased participation in function-focused care activities during hospitalization[5,26] and post hospitalization,

Table 1
Function-focused care for acute care 4-step approach

Four Step FFC-AC-EIT	
Step 1: Environment and policy assessments:	Evaluation of the environment and policy with regard to how they optimize function and physical activity or result in barriers to physical activity. Implement interventions to alter the environment to optimally engage patients in physical activity (clear pathways; set up pleasant walking areas). Incorporate the Mobility Screen and Patient Mobility Rating as a required assessment and incorporate this into the Electronic Medical Record.
Step 2: Education of staff on function-focused care:	Work with champions to provide all nurses and other health care providers on the unit with education about function-focused care, completion of the Mobility Screen and Patient Mobility Rating, elimination of entrenched and inaccurate care approaches (eg, unnecessary tethering of patients with pulse oximetry or oxygen), and motivational techniques for patients to engage them in function and physical activity.
Step 3: Establishing patient goals	Use the findings from the Mobility Screen and Patient Mobility Rating to develop short- (during hospitalization) and long-term patient goals (activity goals for use post discharge). Goals should be focused, such as how long to sit; ambulate; participate in functional activities.
Step 4: Ongoing mentoring and motivating of staff, patients, and families:	Use self-efficacy-based approaches for motivation of staff and patients (performance of the activity; verbal encouragement; role modeling; and elimination of unpleasant sensations). Monitor and evaluate nursing care interactions and provide positive feedback for function-focused care activities. Provide ongoing tidbits that highlight new ways to engage patients in function and physical activity (eg, holiday-based activities, contests to walk to a certain location on the unit). Establish staff contests and reward staff for evidence of function-focused care activities and interactions with patients (eg, a contest for who completes the most Mobility Screens in the previous week).

decreased depression, fear of falling, and delirium, improved function and resilience, increased physical activity, and decreased re-hospitalizations.[2,5,10,26]

FFC-AC is implemented by a Research Nurse Facilitator who works with a stakeholder team and an identified unit champion from each shift to implement the 4 steps of the intervention. The stakeholder meetings (recommended stakeholder team members include a unit manager, hospitalist, rehabilitation therapists, social worker/case manager, clinical nurse specialist, or nurse practitioner) are held monthly and focus on developing unit goals relevant to optimizing function and physical activity of patients and fall prevention using a brainstorming approach. Brainstorming involves having stakeholders identify the challenges to engaging patients in function-focused care activities during their hospital stay.

The first step of FFC-AC involves evaluation of the environment and policies using a checklist to establish if the environment and policies support and encourage participation in function and physical activity among patients. The second step of FFC-AC involves education of staff with a focus on how to evaluate patients for underlying physical capability and ability to transfer and ambulate on the unit using the Mobility Screen and Patient Mobility Rating. These tools were developed by physical therapists and nursing staff[98] and have been used to guide caregivers in setting physical activity goals and expectations for patients. Education, although alone unlikely to change behavior of caregivers, is an important step in the process. Education can be facilitated in formal in-service presentations or by providing written material.

Subsequent to education of staff is the implementation of their new knowledge and assessment skills to set patient goals for function and physical activity while on the unit. This needs to be done with a focus on fall prevention as well. Incorporation of interventions that will strengthen the patient, facilitate safe transfers and toileting (eg, elimination of unnecessary tethers), and avoid leaving the individual alone in a room in an unsafe situation, particularly if the patient has some cognitive impairment are critical.

The last step in the implementation of FFC-AC addresses motivation of patients and staff to engage in function-focused care activities. Motivational techniques involve: (1) use of the previously described self-efficacy-based techniques such as role modeling for staff and patients (eg, walking patients on the unit or self-modeling by posting in the hallway how far the patient walked the previous day); (2) verbal encouragement of patients; (3) positive reinforcement for staff based on direct observation of care interactions with patients and acknowledging and rewarding staff when patients are encouraged and helped to engage in physical activity; (4) having unit-based contests that focus on optimizing physical activity among patients; and (5) providing ongoing "tidbits," which are innovative ideas for how to engage patients in physical activity.

ACUTE CARE FOR ELDERS

The Acute Care for Elders (ACE) model[99] is another approach that has been used to optimize function and physical activity and prevent adverse events such as falls among older hospitalized patients. ACE models focus on 5 components or principles of care including: (1) patient-centered care, which addresses engaging the patient in activities of daily living; (2) mobility; (3) continence; (4) frequent medical review to minimize the adverse effects of treatments; (4) early rehabilitation; and (5) early discharge planning. Based on a systematic review and meta-analysis of 13 randomized controlled and quasi-experimental studies, ACE units were shown to decrease falls and functional decline among hospitalized patients.[100] The specific interventions that seemed to have the greatest impact optimizing function and preventing falls

Table 2
Acute Care for Eelders components to optimize function and physical activity and decrease falls

Adult Care for Elders Component	Activities to Implement
Medical review	• Admission assessment and daily review of medical interventions and impact on the patient • Avoid high-risk medications (eg, psychoactive medications, anticholinergic medications, narcotics) • Remove tethers (eg, intravenous therapy, indwelling catheters, oxygen, pulse oximetry) • Encourage food and fluid, and add supplements as appropriate and needed • Avoid excessive testing (eg, limit blood draws, scans to be used only as needed)
Early rehabilitation	• Assess need for physical therapy at the time of admission not at the time of discharge • Encourage mobility at the highest level of the patient on the unit • Encourage self-care at the highest level of the patient • Provide appropriate assistive devices and individually alter the environment as needed
Patient-centered care	• Provide a physical and cognitive assessment of the patient within 24 h of admission • The assessment should incorporate: mobility, hydration and nutritional status, cognition, functional ability, continence patterns, skin integrity • Encourage standing and ambulation as much as possible • Offer fluids and high protein snacks during the day • Encourage self-care or participation in personal care activities (eg, bathing and dressing) • Avoid leaving the patient alone in a room • Optimize sleep via regulating day and night, reducing noise at night, and increasing physical activity • Re-orient as is appropriate for the patient

included ongoing medical reviews, early rehabilitation, and patient-centered care. Examples of these interventions are given in **Table 2**. Medical review should focus on standardized admission assessment and daily review of high-risk medications, treatments, and procedures. Early rehabilitation included an assessment of the need for physical therapy and engaging the patient in mobility activities and self-care during activities of daily living. Patient-centered care incorporated an assessment of physical function and cognition, including risk of falls and delirium and implementation of interventions to prevent these outcomes. ACE units, although known to be effective in improving functional outcomes, are not a feasible approach to address the large number of hospitalized older adults, a population that is only expected to grow at an unprecedented rate. Thus, there is a need for flexible models that can be implemented on medical and surgical units that serve the majority of hospitalized elders.

CONCLUSION

Despite implementation of both low- and high-tech interventions, there has been no single, effective approach to engaging older adults in physical activity or prevention of falls in acute care settings. Interventions that were effective involved multiple approaches and human interaction investment involving assessment of patients, ongoing interaction to motivate and engage the patient in physical activity and toileting activities, and regular if not ongoing visualization and monitoring of the patient to prevent unsafe independent ambulation and a fall. Easy to implement interventions such as bed alarms give the illusion of providing patients with a falls prevention intervention. Unfortunately, bed alarms have not effectively decreased falls because patients are able to get up and fall before a nurse or other provider is able to help him or her. Moreover, alarms have the negative impact of decreasing physical activity. Some hospitals place alarms on patient beds if the patient scores as being at risk for falls, even if he or she was an independent ambulator. These individuals are needlessly prevented from walking and engaging in physical activity during their hospital stay.

Strategies that may be more effective than alarms for fall prevention should focus around toileting and ongoing supervision/visualization of the patient so that a provider can intervene as the patient initiates movement out of the bed. Helping the individual to transfer or ambulate at this time can prevent a fall as well as optimize function and physical activity. Environmental interventions such as cohorting patients in a single large ward where multiple patients can be visualized at once, clear open hallways to facilitate ambulation, padded floors to prevent injuries in semi-mobile patients, and ongoing use of adjustable height, low beds and access to assistive devices may have some benefit.

Optimization of function and prevention of falls may also be facilitated by decreasing patient risk factors for sedentary activity, deconditioning, and falls. This includes a focus on prevention of delirium through optimal medical management, food and fluid intake, avoidance of polypharmacy, elimination of tethers as soon as possible by discontinuing intravenous administration, indwelling urinary catheters, cardiac monitoring, and other types of interventions that keep patients in beds.

Fall risk assessments tend to place all older adults at risk for falls and thus the completion of these assessments may not maximize nursing staff time in mitigating fall risk. There is a tendency to emphasize the numeric indicator associated with level of risk rather than targeting interventions to the patent's specific risk factors. Furthermore, these assessments often result in the implementation of interventions (eg, bed alarms) that decrease opportunities for physical activity of patients and decrease autonomy and independence. Conversely using human resources and time to engage patients in physical activity and monitor patients in safe environments may be a more effective approach to optimizing physical activity and decreasing falls among older individuals. Families, who provide valuable information about the patient's baseline function, communication strategies, and comfort needs, and nursing assistants, who provide the bulk of direct care, need to be engaged in these efforts. Hospitalists also can support the integration of function-focused, fall prevention strategies into treatment plans and discharge planning.[10]

SUMMARY

Increasing physical activity of patients and decreasing falls is critically important to optimize outcomes for patients and decrease the length of hospital stays. There is no single approach that will effectively assure optimal time spent in physical activity or that a fall will not occur. Multifactorial approaches are needed that focus on the individual risks and challenges within each individual. Consideration should be given to using environment approaches as well as those that deal directly with patients, such as motivational techniques or safety interventions. Although ongoing research tends to focus on testing approaches for how to best increase physical activity and prevent falls, we have sufficient data to support the effectiveness of some approaches and the lack of efficacy of others such as bed alarms. Ongoing research should focus on how to implement effective approaches into real-world settings using appropriate implementation strategies to engage patients and health care providers in the activities and techniques needed to optimize physical activity and decrease falls.

REFERENCES

1. Kalish B, Lee S, Dabney B. Outcomes of inpatient mobilization: a literature review. J Clin Nurs 2013;23:1486–501.
2. Resnick B, Galik E, Enders H, et al. Functional and physical activity of older adults in acute care settings: where we are and where we need to go. J Nurs Care Qual 2011;26(2):169–77.
3. Augustin A, de Quadros A, Sarmento-Leite R. Early sheath removal and ambulation in patients submitted to percutaneous coronary intervention: a randomized clinical trial. Int J Nurs Stud 2010;47:939–45.
4. Chair S, Thompson D, Li S. The effect of ambulation after cardiac catheterization on patient outcomes. J Clin Nurs 2007;16:212–21.
5. Resnick B, Wells C, Galik E, et al. Feasibility and efficacy of function focused care for orthopedic trauma patients. J Trauma Nurs 2016;23(3):144–55.
6. Schweickert W, Pohlman M, Pohlman A, et al. Early physical and occupational therapy in mechanically ventilated, critically ill patients: a randomised controlled trial. Lancet 2009;373:1874–82.
7. Kamel H, Iqbal M, Mogallapu R, et al. Time to ambulation after hip fracture surgery: relation to hospitalization outcomes. J Gerontol A Biol Sci Med Sci 2003; 58:1042–5.
8. Hørdam B, Boolsen MW. Patient involvement in own rehabilitation after early discharge. Scand J Caring Sci 2017;31(4):859–66.
9. Keogh JWL, Pühringer P, Olsen A, et al. Physical activity promotion, beliefs, and barriers among australasian oncology nurses. Oncol Nurs Forum 2017;44(2): 235–45.
10. Boltz M, Resnick B, Chippendale T, et al. Testing a family-centered intervention to promote functional and cognitive recovery in hospitalized older adults. J Am Geriatr Soc 2014;62(12):2398–407.
11. Chandrasekaran S, Ariaretnam S, Tsung J, et al. Early mobilization after total knee replacement reduces the incidence of deep venous thrombosis. ANZ J Surg 2009;79:526–9.
12. Nakao S, Takata S, Uemura H, et al. Early ambulation after total knee arthroplasty prevents patients with osteoarthritis and rheumatoid arthritis from developing postoperative higher levels of D-dimer. J Med Invest 2010;57:146–51.
13. Kurabe S, Ozawa T, Watanabe T, et al. Efficacy and safety of postoperative early mobilization for chronic subdural hematoma in elderly patients. Acta Neurochir 2010;52:1171–4.
14. Langhorne P, Stott D, Knight A, et al. Very early rehabilitation or intensive telemetry after stroke: a pilot randomised trial. Cerebrovasc Dis 2010;29:352–60.
15. Clark D, Lowman J, Griffin R, et al. Effectiveness of an early mobilization protocol in a trauma and burns intensive care unit: a retrospective cohort study. Phys Ther 2013;93(2):186–96.

16. Fisher SR, Galloway R, Kuo YF, et al. Pilot study examining the association between ambulatory activity and falls among hospitalized older adults. Arch Intern Med 2011;92:2090–2.
17. Castillo R, MacKenzie E, Archer K, et al. Evidence of beneficial effect of physical therapy after lower-extremity trauma. Arch Phys Med Rehabil 2008;89:1873–9.
18. Needham D, Korupolu R, Zanni J, et al. Early physical medicine and rehabilitation for patients with acute respiratory failure: a quality improvement project. Arch Phys Med Rehabil 2010;91:536–42.
19. Bailey P, Thomsen GE, Spuhler VJ, et al. Early activity is feasible and safe in respiratory failure patients. Crit Care Med 2007;35(1):139–45.
20. Thomsen GE, Snow GL, Rodriguez L, et al. Patients with respiratory failure increase ambulation after transfer to an intensive care unit where early activity is a priority. Crit Care Med 2008;36(4):119–1124.
21. Hopkins R, Spuhler VJ. Strategies for promoting early activity in critically ill mechanically ventilated patients. AACN Adv Crit Care 2009;20:277–89.
22. Burtin C, Clerckx B, Robbeets C, et al. Early exercise in critically ill patients enhances short term functional recovery. Crit Care Med 2009;37:2499–505.
23. Cumming T, Thrift A, Collier J, et al. Very early mobilization after stroke fast-tracks return to walking: further results from the phase II AVERT randomized controlled trial. Stroke 2011;42:153–8.
24. Padula C, Hughes C, Baumhover L. Impact of nurse-driven mobility protocol on functional decline in hospitalized older adults. J Nurs Care Qual 2009;24:325–31.
25. Boltz M, Resnick B, Capezuti E, et al. Functional decline in hospitalized older adults: can nursing make a difference? Geriatr Nurs 2012;33(4):272–9.
26. Boltz M, Chippendale T, Resnick B, et al. Testing family-centered, function-focused care in hospitalized persons with dementia. Neurodegener Dis Manag 2015;5(3):203–15.
27. Brown CJ, Redden DT, KFlood KL, et al. The underrecognized epidemic of low mobility during hospitalization of older adults. J Am Geriatr Soc 2009;57(9):1660–7.
28. Edmonds C, Smith H. Observational pilot study of physical activity on an acute older person's unit. Age Ageing 2014;43(Supplement 1):i33.
29. Fisher S, Goodwin J, Protas E, et al. Ambulatory activity of older adults hospitalized with acute medical illness. J Am Geriatr Soc 2011;59(1):91–5.
30. Kuys S, Dolecka U, Guard A. Activity level of hospital medical inpatients: an observational study. Arch Gerontol Geriat 2012;55(2):417–22.
31. McRae P, Peel N, Walker P, et al. Geriatric syndromes in individuals admitted to vascular and urology surgical units. J Am Geriatr Soc 2014;62:1105–9.
32. Zisberg A, Sahadmi E, Gur-Yaish N, et al. Hospital associated functional decline: the role of hospitalization processes beyond individual risk factors. J Am Geriatr Soc 2015;63(1):55–62.
33. Zisberg A, Shadmi E, Sinoff G, et al. Low mobility during hospitalization and functional decline in older adults. J Am Geriatr Soc 2011;59:266–73.
34. News Report Column. Nurses fall short in promoting physical activity to patients. Aust Nurs Midwifery J 2017;24(10):10.
35. Tobiano G, Marshall A, Bucknall T, et al. Activities patients and nurses undertake to promote patient participation. J Nurs Scholarsh 2016;48(4):362–70.
36. Brown CJ, Peel C, Bamman MM, et al. Exercise program implementation proves not feasible during acute care hospitalization. J Rehabil Res Dev 2006;43(7):939–46.

37. Brown CJ, Williams BR, Woodby LL, et al. Barriers to mobility during hospitalization from the perspective of the patient, their nurses and physicians. J Hosp Med 2007;2:305–31.

38. Buttery AK, Martin FC. Knowledge, attitudes and intentions about participation in physical activity of older post acute hospital inpatients. Physiotherapy 2009; 95(3):192–8.

39. Burdick D, Rosenblatt A, Samus QM, et al. Predictors of functional impairment in residents of assisted living facilities: the Maryland Assisted Living Study. J Gerontol A Biol Sci Med Sci 2005;60(2):258–64.

40. Wakefield B, Holman J. Functional trajectories associated with hospitalization in older adults. West J Nurs Res 2007;29(2):161–77.

41. Boltz M, Capezuti E, Bowar-Ferres S, et al. Hospital nurses' perception of the geriatric nurse practice environment. J Nurs Scholarsh 2008;40(3):282–9.

42. Lee D, Shook R, Drenowatz C, et al. Physical activity and sarcopenic obesity: definition, assessment, prevalence and mechanism. Future Sci OA 2016;2: 127–31.

43. Batsis J, Zbehlik A, Pidgeon D, et al. Dynapenic obesity and the effect on long-term physical function and quality of life: data from the osteoarthritis initiative. BMC Geriatr 2015;15:118. Available at: https://www.ncbi.nlm.nih.gov/pubmed/26449277.

44. Dermody G, Kovach CR. Nurses' experience with and perception of barriers to promoting mobility in hospitalized older adults: a descriptive study. J Gerontol Nurs 2017;43(11):22–9.

45. Jette E, Brown R, Collette N, et al. Physical therapists' management of patients in the acute care setting: an observational study. Phys Ther 2010;89(11): 1158–75.

46. Lenze EJ, Miller MD, Dew MA, et al. Subjective health measures and acute treatment outcomes in geriatric depression. Int J Geriatr Psychiatry 2001;16(12): 1149–55.

47. de Morton N, Keating J, Jeffs K. Exercise for acutely hospitalised older medical patients. Cochrane Database Syst Rev 2007;(1):CD005955.

48. Nolan J, Thomas S. Targeted individual exercise programmes for older medical patients are feasible, and may change hospital and patient outcomes: a service improvement project. BMC Health Serv Res 2008;8:250.

49. Balas MC, Vasilevskis EE, Olsen KM, et al. Effectiveness and safety of the awakening and breathing coordination, delirium monitoring/management, and early exercise/mobility bundle. Crit Care Med 2014;42(5):1024–36.

50. Leditschke A, Green M, Irvine J, et al. What are the barriers to mobilizing intensive care patients? Cardiopulm Phys Ther J 2012;23(1):26–9.

51. Palese A. Hospital acquired functional decline in older patients cared for in acute medical wards and predictors: findings from a multicentre longitudinal study. Geriatr Nurs 2016;37(3):192–9.

52. Tucker SJ, Carr LJ. Translating physical activity evidence to hospital settings. Clin Nurse Spec 2016;30(4):208–15.

53. So C, Pierluissi E. Attitudes and expectations regarding exercise in the hospital of hospitalized older adults: a qualitative study. J Am Geriatr Soc 2012;60: 713–8.

54. de Morton NA, Keating JL, Berlowitz DJ, et al. Additional exercise does not change hospital or patient outcomes in older medical patients: a controlled clinical trial. Aust J Physiother 2007;53(2):105–11.

55. Davis E, Biddinson J, Cohen-Mansfield J. Hip fracture rehabilitation in persons with dementia: how much should we invest? Ann Longterm Care 2008;16:7–10.

56. Huusko T, Karppi P, Avikainen V, et al. Randomised, clinically controlled trial of intensive geriatric rehabilitation in patients with hip fracture: subgroup analysis of patients with dementia. Br Med J 2000;321(7269):1107–11.

57. Mittmann N, Seng S, Pisterzi L, et al. Nursing workload associated with hospital patient care. Disease Management & Health Outcomes 2008;16(1):53–61.

58. Williams H, Harris R, Turner-Stokes L. Work sampling: a quantitative analysis of nursing activity in a neuro-rehabilitation setting. J Adv Nurs 2009;65(10):2097–107.

59. Doherty-King B, Yoon J, Pecanac K, et al. Frequency and duration of nursing care related to older patient mobility. J Nurs Scholarsh 2014;46(1):20–7.

60. Boltz M, Resnick B, Capezuti E, et al. Function-focused activity and changes in physical function in Chinese and non-Chinese hospitalized older adults. Rehabil Nurs 2011;36(6):233–40.

61. Shever LL, Titler M, Dochterman J, et al. Patterns of nursing intervention use across 6 days of acute care hospitalization for three older patient populations. Int J Nurs Terminol Classif 2007;18(1):18–29.

62. Volpato S, Onder G, Cavalieri M, et al. Characteristics of nondisabled older patients developing new disability associated with medical illnesses and hospitalization. J Gen Intern Med 2007;22(5):668–74.

63. Resnick B, Wells C, Brotemarkle R, et al. Exposure to therapy of older patients with trauma and factors that influence therapy opportunities. Phys Ther 2014;94(1):40–51.

64. Inouye SK, Brown CJ, Tinetti ME. Medicare nonpayment, hospital falls, and unintended consequences. N Engl J Med 2009;360:2390–3.

65. Boltz M, Resnick B, Capezuti E, et al. Activity restriction vs. self-direction: hospitalised older adults' response to fear of falling. Int J Older People Nurs 2014;9(1):44–53.

66. Shuman C, Liu J, Montie M, et al. Patient perceptions and experiences with falls during hospitalization and after discharge. Appl Nurs Res 2016;31:79–85.

67. Bouldin ED, Andresen EM, Dunton NE, et al. Falls among adult patients hospitalized in the United States: prevalence and trends. J Patient Saf 2013;9(1):13–7.

68. Miake-Lyke IM, Hempel S, Ganz DA, et al. Inpatient fall prevention programs as a patient safety strategy: a systematic review. Ann Intern Med 2013;158(5 pt 2):390–6.

69. Oliver D, Healey F, Haines TP. Preventing falls and fall related injuries in hospitals. Clin Geriatr Med 2010;26(4):645–92.

70. Alzheimer's Association. Alzheimer's disease facts and figures. Alzheimer's Dement 2016;12(4):100–1.

71. Phelan EA, Borson S, Grothaus L, et al. Association of incident dementia with hospitalizations. J Am Med Assoc 2012;307:165–70.

72. Chen X, Nguyen H, Shen Q, et al. Characteristics associated with recurrent falls among the elderly within aged care wards in a tertiary hospital: the effect of cognitive impairment. Arch Gerontol Geriatr 2011;53:e183–6.

73. Haines TP, Hill AM, Hill KD. Patient education to prevent falls among older hospital inpatients: a randomized controlled trial. Arch Intern Med 2011;171:516–24.

74. Hughes C, Kneebone I, Jones F, et al. A theoretical and empirical review of psychological factors associated with falls-related psychological concerns in community-dwelling older people. Int Psychogeriatr 2015;27(7):1071–87.

75. Kröpelin T, Neyens J, Halfens R, et al. Fall determinants in older long-term care residents with dementia: a systematic review. Int Psychogeriatr 2013;25(4): 549–63.

76. Taylor M, Delbaere K, Lord S, et al. Neuropsychological, physical, and functional mobility measures associated with falls in cognitively impaired older adults. J Gerontol A Biol Sci Med Sci 2014;69(8):987–95.

77. Noublanche F, Simon R, Decavel F, et al. Falls prediction in acute care units: preliminary results from a prospective cohort study. J Am Geriatr Soc 2014;62(8): 1605–6.

78. Hitcho EB, Krauss MJ, Birge S. Characteristics and circumstances of falls in a hospital setting: a prospective analysis. J Gen Intern Med 2004;19:732–9.

79. Chan DKY, Sherrington CLS, Finch CF, et al. Key issues to consider and innovative ideas on fall prevention in the geriatric department of a teaching hospital. Australas J Ageing 2018;37(2):140–3.

80. Hempel S, Newberry S, Wang Z, et al. Hospital fall prevention: a systematic review of implementation, components, adherence, and effectiveness. J Am Geriatr Soc 2013;61(4):483–94.

81. Cameron ID, Gillepspie LD, Robertson MC. Interventions for preventing falls in older people in care facilities and hospitals. Cochrane Database Syst Rev 2012;(12):CD005465.

82. Gillespie LD, Robertson MC, Gilespie WJ. Interventions for preventing falls in older people living in the community. Cochrane Database Syst Rev 2012;(9):CD007146.

83. Shorr RI, Chandler AM, Mion LC, et al. Effects of an intervention to increase bed alarm use to prevent falls in hospitalized patients: a cluster randomized trial. Ann Intern Med 2012;157(10):692–9.

84. Barker AL, Morello RT, Ayton DR, et al. Acceptability of the 6-PACK falls prevention program: a pre-implementation study in hospitals participating in a cluster randomized controlled trial. PLoS One 2017;12(2):e0172005.

85. Anderson O, Boshier PR, Hanna GB. Interventions designed to prevent healthcare bed-related injuries in patients. Cochrane Database Syst Rev 2012;(1):CD008931.

86. Wolf KH, Hetzer K, zu Schwabedissen HM, et al. Development and pilot study of a bed-exit alarm based on a body-worn accelerometer. Z Gerontol Geriatr 2013; 46(8):727–33.

87. Hardin SR, Dienemann J, Rudisill P, et al. Inpatient fall prevention: use of in-room webcams. J Patient Saf 2013;9(1):29–35.

88. Guarascio-Howard L. Examination of wireless technology to improve nurse communication, response time to bed alarms, and patient safety. HERD 2011; 4(2):109–20.

89. Lohse GR, Leopold SS, Theiler S, et al. Systems-based safety intervention: reducing falls with injury and total falls on an orthopaedic ward. J Bone Joint Surg Am 2012;94:1217–22.

90. Cozart HC. Environmental effects on incidence of falls in the hospitalized elderly. 2009 [Doctoral Dissertation, Texas Women's University]. Available at: https://twu-ir.tdl.org/handle/11274/143.

91. Fleury J, Lee SM. The social ecological model and physical activity in African American women. Am J Community Psychol 2006;1:1–8.

92. Gregson J, Foerster S, Orr R, et al. System, environment and policy changes: using the Social Ecological Model as a framework for evaluating nutrition education and social marketing programs with low income audiences. J Nutr Educ 2003;33:S4–15.
93. Bandura A. Self-efficacy in changing societies. New York: Cambridge University Press; 1995.
94. Bandura A. Self-efficacy: the exercise of control. New York: W.H. Freeman and Company.; 1997.
95. Bandura A. Health promotion by social cognitive means. Health Educ Behav 2004;31(2):143–64.
96. Burkett T, Hippensteel N, Penrod J, et al. Pilot testing of the function focused care intervention on an acute care trauma unit. Geriatr Nurs 2013;34(3):241–6.
97. Galik E, Resnick B, Pretzer-Aboff I. Knowing what makes them tick: motivating cognitively impaired older adults to participate in restorative care. International Journal of Nursing Practice 2009;15(1):48–55.
98. Resnick B, Galik E, Boltz M, et al, editors. Implementing restorative care nursing in all setting. 2nd edition. New York: Springer; 2011.
99. Resnick B. Restorative care and motivating older adults to engage in these activities. Video Press University of Maryland School of Medicine; 2001. Available at: http://www.functionfocusedcare.com.
100. Fox MT, Persaud M, Maimets I, et al. Effectiveness of acute geriatric unit care using acute care for elders components: a systematic review and meta analysis. J Am Geriatr Soc 2012;60:2237–45.

Outcomes of Patient-Engaged Video Surveillance on Falls and Other Adverse Events

Patricia A. Quigley, PhD, MPH, MS[a],*, Lisbeth Votruba, MSN, RN[b],
Jill Kaminski, MS[b]

KEYWORDS

- Surveillance • Falls • Fall prevention • Outcomes • Patient engagement
- TeleSitting

KEY POINTS

- Patient-engaged video surveillance is effective in reducing falls, room elopement, and line, tube, or drain dislodgement.
- Formal, trained 24-hour monitoring is more effective in reducing falls than sitters, bed alarms, and purposeful rounding.
- Constant observation and individualized patient interaction decreases the burden of staff response to false alarms and alarm fatigue.
- Across all adult age groups, patients respond positively to patient-engaged video surveillance.
- Data and fact-based outcomes of patient-engaged video surveillance on falls and other adverse events are explored.

INTRODUCTION

The continued burden of hospital-acquired adverse events on patient loss of function and life requires that all health care organizations stop surveillance practices that create a false sense of safety. This article summarizes current knowledge about patient surveillance integrated into clinical practice and patient safety outcomes in the hospital setting. Evidence of the efficiency and effectiveness of traditional surveillance system measures such as call bells, bed alarms, and intentional rounding lacks methodologic rigor. The integration of such technology for all patients, irrespective of

Disclosures: P.A. Quigley: Independent Contractor and Fall Prevention Expert, AvaSure, LLC. L. Votruba: VP of Clinical Quality and Innovation at AvaSure, LLC. J. Kaminski: Clinical Data and Systems Analyst at AvaSure, LLC.
[a] Nurses Consultant, LLC, 6297 25th Street North, St Petersburg, FL 33702, USA; [b] AvaSure, LLC, 5801 Safety Drive, Belmont, MI 49306, USA
* Corresponding author.
E-mail address: pquigley1@tampabay.rr.com

geriatric.theclinics.com

cognitive status, increases unnecessary burden to the nursing workforce and fails to individualize patient safety prevention. Health care leaders, in efforts to fast track patient safety improvement, are investing in patient-engaged video surveillance (PEVS) technology that ensures patient and family engagement, patient care privacy, individualized care planning, and workforce safety. This article presents the results of continuous PEVS on patient falls, room elopement, and line, tube, or drain dislodgement across 71 hospitals between June 1, 2017, and May 31, 2018.

SLOW PROGRESS IN REDUCING PATIENT HARM

The slow progress in reducing the burden of hospital-acquired harm requires that organizations must commit to transforming patient safety practices.[1] The inpatient population's vulnerability to harm has increased, and interdisciplinary teams fail to implement reliable patient safety interventions based on vulnerability. In 2010, 45% of the inpatient hospital population in the United States was 65 years of age and older, among whom 19% were ages 75 to 84 years of age and 9% were 85 years of age and older. These findings should compel all organizations to implement patient safety programs based on increased vulnerability to hospital-acquired harm that results in loss of function or loss of life. For example, falls in persons 85 years of age and older are the leading cause of unintentional injury death.[2] Levant and associates[2] urged organizations to intentionally correct root causes of harm, which is best achieved when root causes are observed and reported.

Since 2010, Centers for Medicare & Medicaid Services have provided funding for health organizations to implement patient safety practices that decrease patient harm, as monitored by scorecards reported by the Agency for Healthcare Research and Quality.[3] A new national goal for 2017 was to decrease harm 20% overall by 2019. The Agency for Healthcare Research and Quality in 2018 released the newest scorecard data on gains in patient safety by reducing hospital-acquired conditions. In 2015 and 2016, the results reported an 8% decline in all hospital-acquired conditions.[4] It is well-known that falls in hospitals are high volume and high cost. Prior research has confirmed that 3% to 20% of patients in hospitals fall at least once[5] and of those who fall, 30% to 51% are injured.[6] In 2017, The Joint Commission reviewed a total of 805 sentinel alerts. Falls were the second highest reported sentinel alert (n = 114). From 2014 to the second quarter of 2017, fall sentinel events were the third top reported harm event in the nation, preceded only by unintended retention of a foreign body, and by wrong patient, wrong site, or wrong procedures.[7] The slow reduction of adverse conditions, particularly falls—and, ultimately, injurious falls— confirms that current practices are ineffective. Data do not exist on harm to patients owing to line, tube, or drain dislodgements or eloping from their room.

AVAILABLE KNOWLEDGE

Keeping patients safe in their rooms within clinical units is still predominately the responsibility of nursing staff. For decades, nurses have relied on traditional surveillance methods to proactively meet patient needs: hourly rounding, patient-activated call lights, and movement-initiated alarms. Recently, these methods have been supplemented by cameras installed in rooms in the intensive care unit or emergency department psychiatry holding areas, allowing anyone at a nurses' station to observe patients. The ineffectiveness of these traditional interventions is confirmed by a limited number of published studies and the epidemic of harm still occurring in hospitals.

Evidence reviews report that hourly rounding leads to improved patient satisfaction, decreased fear, improved perceptions in nursing care, decreased call light use, and decreased aggregated fall rates.[8] However, these studies lack methodologic rigor in the form of inconsistent reporting of the quantity, quality, and reliability of rounding. The association with decreased fall rates is not linked to the specific type of fall prevention intervention, nor is it aligned with the specific type of fall (eg, an accidental or anticipated physiologic fall).

Both patient use of call lights, a universal tool, as well as nurse responsiveness have been linked to patient care satisfaction and safety. Tzeng and colleagues[9] reported a relationship between faster call light response time and decreased fall rates and injurious fall rates. The average call light response time across 4 hospitals was 13 minutes and 18 seconds. The hospital with the longest response time was 17 minutes and 27 seconds. Patients can successfully exit a bed or chair and fall during this time interval. Among patients included in their study, 9.93% of patients admitted had altered mental status and could not reliably use a call light. The total fall rate was 4.08 per 1000 patient-days. Total injurious falls was 0.91 per 1000 patient-days. The percent of patients 65 and older was 35.93%.

Movement alarms are among the most commonly used fall prevention strategies in hospitals.[10] In research on these alarms, the most commonly used outcome measure is number of falls,[11] percent of fallers,[12] or fall rates.[12,13] Studies on patients rescued from experiencing a fall, and on the reduction in falls, fallers, or fall rates are very limited. Furthermore, there are no published studies on the timeliness of nursing staff response to patients' activated alarms.

PATIENT-ENGAGED VIDEO SURVEILLANCE

Video surveillance is a common intervention method used to monitor people and processes throughout industries. Use in hospitals has predominately been in emergency room holding areas and intensive care units. PEVS is a more interactive form of video surveillance, with dedicated and trained staff using a hospital workstation to monitor multiple patients simultaneously. Through a 2-way audio communication system, a monitoring staff member verbally engages with the patient. Monitoring staff become familiar with patients' behavioral patterns and can proactively intervene before patients attempt risky behaviors such as getting out of bed without assistance. Monitoring staff can verbally redirect patients, contact caregivers, and trigger an alarm if necessary. Patients are selected for PEVS based on bedside clinical assessment. Patients most at risk for falls and other adverse events often have an impaired mental status. Published articles on PEVS show effective outcomes in decreasing overall fall and injury rates. Preventing falls through the selection and observation of the most at-risk patients impacts overall hospital and/or care unit fall and injury rates.[14-18] These studies also show effective outcomes in cost savings through reducing falls, falls with injuries, and one-to-one sitter costs. Although the outcomes are consistent, the sample sizes of patients enrolled in PEVS has remained small, limited by the number of purchased monitors (ie, Cournan and colleagues[18] reported only 15 patient monitors with 1 monitor tech in a 115-bed hospital). Data collection was dependent on manual data collection from monitor staff. There have been no studies measuring the timeliness of rescue (ie, clinical response time to PEVS alarms).

Design

A descriptive study based on large-scale program evaluation data was conducted to answer the following research questions:

1. What is the age distribution of the adult population enrolled in PEVS? What is the duration of PEVS?

2. Do trends in verbal patient engagement, alarm rate, and alarm response time vary by age group?
3. Does the rate of adverse events (fall, room elopement, and line, tube, or drain dislodgement) vary by age group?
4. Do differences exist by patient age, monitor staff engagement, and response time, and do these differences impact fall rates?
5. What is the potential cost savings difference between PEVs and 1:1 sitter usage?

Methods

Across all 71 hospitals, the same PEVS system was implemented. Data were collected from the national data reporting system. The program implemented was AvaSys®, a telehealth solution that includes a monitoring device, which is either permanently installed or mobile, in the patient's room. AvaSys transmitted an audio–video feed across each hospital's secured wireless network to a workstation where 1 trained monitoring staff member interacted with up to 16 patients at once. The primary bedside nurse selected appropriate patients for PEVS, based on nursing judgment and hospital-specific policies, and worked with the monitor staff to set up and individualize PEVS. Patients were deemed high risk for an adverse event based on factors such as altered mental status, acuity, agitation, and impaired mobility. During surveillance, the monitoring staff learned the patient's behaviors and verbally engaged the patient before adverse events occurred. The bedside caregivers were also able to request a virtual privacy screen during personal patient care. In the case of an urgent or emergent observed behavior, a PEVS alarm was triggered. The top 3 adverse events prevented were assisted and unassisted falls, room elopement, and line, tube, or drain dislodgement.

Measures

Data collection

Data were captured automatically from PEVS into a national database as video monitoring staff observed and intervened. The data were stored securely via cloud for ease of data export and analysis with RStudio®. The 71 participating hospitals in this study were selected based on the presence of intervention data logging and patient age. All participating hospitals had an executed agreement allowing for the analysis and publication of aggregate data. On a monthly basis, AvaSure, LLC (Belmont, MI), securely exported raw data from the hospitals' servers. This data did not contain protected health information, as defined by the Safe Harbor method.[19] The data were then aggregated to provide program metrics and national benchmarking for subscribers.

Key Metrics

Monitoring staff software interactions were automatically captured to provide the following patient engagement metrics.

- Verbal interventions: occurrences of monitoring staff using the talk button to speak directly to patients.
- PEVS alarm: occurrences of monitoring staff activating the alarm.
- Alarm response time: a measure of the amount of time elapsed between activation and deactivation of the PEVS alarm.

The software also allowed monitoring staff to report which of their interventions likely avoided an adverse event, with a brief description of the circumstances. The top 3 reported adverse events included the following.

- Fall: When a fall is observed, monitoring staff immediately report the fall event witnessed and whether it was an assisted or unassisted fall. They do not report falls with injury, because monitoring staff are not qualified and do not have enough information to determine if an injury has occurred with a fall.
- Elopement: Monitoring staff report when a patient leaves the threshold of his room. They do not, however, report when a patient leaves the hospital building because they are not able to observe outside of the patient's room.
- Line, tube, or drain dislodged: Monitoring staff report if a patient dislodges a medical device such as a peripheral intravenous catheter, Foley catheter, or nasal cannula.

The adverse event rate is calculated by dividing the number of adverse events by days of surveillance on PEVS and multiplying by 1000. This rate is consistent with national standards for the reporting of fall rates per 1000 patient-days.

Results

Between July 1, 2017, and May 31, 2018 there were 15,021 patients 18 years of age or older; these patients were monitored for a total of 942,482 hours (39,270 patient-days). The average length of surveillance was 62.7 hours (**Table 1**). On average, monitoring staff talked to patients 15.8 times per patient day (616,006 total verbal interventions) and activated 1.6 alarms per patient day (61,003 total alarms). The average alarm response time was 15.8 seconds (**Table 2**). The observed reported adverse events included a total of 59 falls witnessed by monitoring staff during PEVS: 44 (75%) were unassisted falls and 15 (25%) were assisted. None of the patients fell more than once; thus, the number of patients who fell was 59. Adults younger than 65 years old were more likely to fall during surveillance than patients 65 years or older ($P = .002$). The oldest age group ($\geq$85 years old) experienced the lowest rate of falls per 1000 days of surveillance (0.38). There were 106 incidents of dislodgement that occurred. The oldest age group also experienced the lowest rate of line, tube, or drain dislodgements per 1000 days of surveillance (2.30). Twenty-seven patients eloped from their rooms. Patients between the ages of 65 and 84 years had the lowest elopement rate per 1000 patient-days (0.42; **Table 3**). The overall fall rate was 1.50 falls per 1000 days of surveillance, and the unassisted fall rate was 1.12 unassisted falls per 1000 days of surveillance. The number of room elopements and the number of line, tube, or drain dislodgements was also reported per 1000 days of surveillance (**Table 4**).

Patients who experienced a fall had 20.5 verbal interventions per patient day, compared with 15.7 verbal interventions per patient day for those who did not fall ($P = .0005$). The falling group also had a higher number of alarms than the nonfalling

Table 1				
Patient-engaged video surveillance patient age and use				
Factors	Age (y)			Total
	18–64	65–84	≥85	
No. of patients	5173	6393	3455	15,021
Hours	359,584	395,392	187,506	942,482
No. of patient-days	14,983	16,475	7813	39,270
Length of surveillance (h/d)	69.5/2.9	61.8/2.5	54.3/2.3	62.7/2.6

Data collected from June 1, 2017, to May 31, 2018 from 71 hospitals.

Table 2
Patient engagement interventions

	Age (y)			
	18–64	65–84	≥85	Total
No. of patients	5173	6393	3455	15,021
No. of verbal interventions	223,207	270,869	121,930	616,006
No. of PEVS alarms	21,081	26,113	13,809	61,003
Verbal interventions per patient-day	14.9	16.4	15.6	15.8
PEVS alarms per patient-day	1.4	1.6	1.8	1.6
Average PEVS alarm response time (s)	17.7	14.8	14.7	15.8

Abbreviation: PEVS, patient-engaged video surveillance.
Data collected from June 1, 2017, to May 31, 2018 from 71 hospitals.

group, namely, 2.38 and 1.55, respectively ($P = .01$). PEVS alarm response time for patients who experienced unassisted falls was slower at 19.2 seconds, as compared with the aggregate response time of 15.8 seconds ($P = .07$).

There were 453 annualized full-time equivalents that would be required to provide 942,482 hours of surveillance by the traditional one-to-one sitter method. With PEVS provided at a monitoring staff to patient ratio of 1:12, the total number of required full-time equivalents is reduced by 92% to 38 full-time equivalents. The actual cost savings are contingent on the hourly wages of the one-to-one sitters and monitoring staff.

There were no differences in alarm or verbal intervention rates between the 3 age groups. Somewhat less engagement from monitoring staff, as measured by verbal interventions and alarm rates, was noted for patients 65 years old or younger. Bedside caregivers were noted to respond more slowly to alarms from patients in the youngest age group.

Discussion

Over 1 year, clinical nurses from 71 hospitals selected 15,021 patients they believed were at greatest risk for falls and other adverse events. Studying the outcomes of PEVS on this group of high-risk patients gives a new window into understanding the effectiveness of PEVS. Estimating the anticipated fall rate had the 15,021 patients

Table 3
Monitoring staff reported adverse events

	Age (y)			
	18–64	65–84	≥85	Total
No. of patients	5173	6393	3455	15,021
Total falls	34	22	3	59
Unassisted falls	26	16	2	44
Assisted falls	8	6	1	15
Elopements (from patient room)	14	7	6	27
Line, tube, or drains dislodged	40	48	18	106
Total adverse events	122	99	30	251

Data collected from June 1, 2017, to May 31, 2018 from 71 hospitals.

Table 4
Adverse event rates per 1000 days of surveillance

	Age (y)			
	18–64	65–84	≥85	Total
Total falls per 1000 days of surveillance	2.27	1.34	0.38	1.50
Assisted falls per 1000 days of surveillance	0.53	0.36	0.13	0.38
Unassisted falls per 1000 days of surveillance	1.74	0.97	0.26	1.12
Elopements per 1000 days of surveillance	0.93	0.42	0.77	0.69
Line, tube, or drains dislodged per 1000 days of surveillance	2.67	2.91	2.30	2.70

Data collected from June 1, 2017, to May 31, 2018 from 71 hospitals.

received traditional fall prevention interventions without PEVS would be difficult because the same protocol for patient selection was not used across all the hospitals. The fact that the overall fall rate was only 1.50 falls per 1000 days of surveillance demonstrates the effectiveness of PEVS. It is especially encouraging to see that the fall rate in the oldest age group (≥85 years of age), which is most vulnerable to fall injury, was only 0.38 falls per 1000 days of surveillance.

The findings of our study should impress on all organizations the confirmed positive contribution that innovative technology is making on patient safety for the adult population. Traditional fall prevention programs are failing to prevent falls, and progress toward reducing falls in an aging patient population has been slow. Our study shows that continuous observation and timeliness of response are key factors in preventing falls. These results also support population-based selection criteria based on clinical risk factors for falls and injury risk, not merely a score on a fall risk screening tool. Health care organizations should implement policies for patient selection based on vulnerability, such as protecting those 85 years of age or older, with confusion or impulsivity from falls. Then clinical training programs for constant observation and patient engagement would be population specific.

Our study adds to the body of evidence suggesting that timeliness of response is a key factor in preventing falls. It was noted that patients who fell while on PEVS had a statistically significant longer alarm response time than patients who did not fall while on PEVS (19.2 seconds and 15.8 seconds, respectively). This means that just 3.4 seconds can make all the difference in rescuing a patient from a fall. The results of our study provide original data on how quickly a patient can experience a fall. Even within an extremely rapid alarm response time of seconds, fall events did occur.

Again, compare this outcome with the work of Tzeng and colleagues,[9] whose data were discussed elsewhere in this article and demonstrated a relationship between faster call light response time and decreased fall rates and injurious fall rates. However, their call light response time average, of 13 minutes and 18 seconds, is more than 10 times longer than responses times in PEVS alarms reporting. Their study also reported a higher fall rate than the reported PEVS fall rate (4.08/1000 patient-days and injurious falls 0.91/1000 patient-days). The fact that call light response time averages are more than 10 times longer than PEVS alarm response time averages should be a significant consideration for organizations entrusted with patient care and safety. The results of our study add evidence suggesting that timeliness of response is a key factor in preventing falls.

Interestingly, it was also noted that, although verbal interventions and alarms were close to the same rate in the 65 to 84 year old range and the 85 years and older age range, there were far fewer falls in the older age group ($P = .008$; **Fig. 1**. This finding

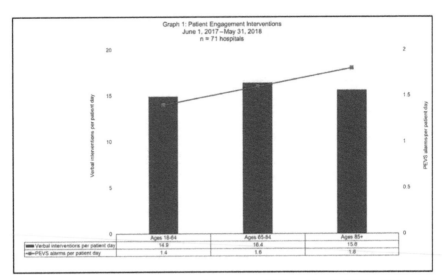

Fig. 1. Patient engagement interventions from June 1, 2017, to May 31, 2018 at 71 hospitals. PEVS, patient engaged video surveillance.

may indicate that older adults take longer to get to a standing position,[20] allowing more time for nursing staff to respond and prevent the fall. However, this finding does not decrease the need for timeliness of response to alarms in preventing patient falls. Indeed, see Jones and colleagues,[20] who established age-specific values, based on biomechanical research and quantified within 30 seconds, for adults of varying ages completing cycles of standing from a sitting position and sitting back down—referred to as sit-to-stand cycles. The time for each cycle provides insight into how quickly a fall can occur from a chair. An older adult between the ages of 65 and 69 can complete between 11 and 16 sit-to-stand cycles within 30 seconds (taking 2.72 seconds for each sit-to-stand cycle, and 1.88 seconds for each stand-to-sit cycle). A person between 85 and 89 years of age can perform 8 to 13 sit-to-stand cycles within 30 seconds (for a slower individual, 3.75 seconds for 8 cycles in 30 seconds; or for a faster individual, 2.30 seconds for 13 cycles in 30 seconds). It would take a person more seconds to transition from lying to sitting to standing, or fewer seconds if he were to roll out of bed onto the floor.

Considering this discussion, our results showing that PEVS increases rapid nurse response are significant for organizations seeking to implement patient safety programs based on increased vulnerability. PEVS promotes rapid nurse response because, when monitor technicians see an urgent or emergent patient need, they activate the PEVS alarm. Used only when patients are in imminent danger of an adverse event, the PEVS alarm is recognized by unit nursing staff as signaling an urgent need and thus elicits a quick response within seconds to the bedside.

The results of our study also showcase the variations in patient safety for the oldest of patients—patients who are 85 years of age or older. Data showed that monitoring staff used slightly fewer verbal interventions and slightly more PEVS alarms for the patient population 85 years of age or older—a patient population with a higher likelihood of experiencing increased confusion and/or difficulty hearing. If monitor staff decreased their verbal interventions for these reasons, perhaps even per nursing staff instruction, monitor staff would have a higher incidence of needing to call nursing staff to the patient's bedside with an alarm. This factor could perhaps account for the findings of our study showing that bedside caregivers are quicker to respond to older patient populations. Responding quickly to older patients is a best practice in age-specific fall and injury prevention that is protective. Our findings confirm that nursing staff implemented age-specific care.

These findings become critically important when viewed alongside other data. For example, consider the original research conducted by Levant and colleagues,[2] in 2015, who explored the epidemiology of the aging of the inpatient hospital population from 2000 to 2010, with special focus on persons 85 year of age and older. They found that, in 2010, 45% of the inpatient hospital population in the United States was 65 years of age and older, among whom 19% were ages 75 to 84 years old and 9% were at least 84 year old. Furthermore, consider that falls are the leading cause of unintentional injury deaths in adults 85 and older. These findings should compel all organizations to implement patient safety programs based on increased vulnerability.

Last, clinical decision-making tools within organizations should be further differentiated for the selection of sitter use versus purposeful rounding with PEVS, because the indications may be redundant for select populations. The need exists for comparison of PEVS, sitter use, and/or purposeful rounding. Organizations should define clear selection criteria and training programs for the nursing staff.

Limitations

One limitation to point out is that, during PEVS implementation, all hospitals received the same implementation training program for monitoring staff and nursing staff support. However, hospitals were allowed to modify their protocol for patient selection and enrollment. For example, 1 hospital implementation committee could select to enroll neurologic and rehabilitation patients, whereas another hospital could select to enroll medical/surgical and orthopedic units. Control for unit types and acuity was not possible. Therefore, the analysis to risk adjust based on acuity was not possible.

A second limitation in our study is in regard to the top 3 observed adverse events reported. In the case of room elopement and line, tube, or drain dislodgement, no comparison of national rates can be made between organizations using PEVS and those not using PEVS because these adverse events are not reported to national public comparison databases.

A third limitation in our study is estimating the anticipated fall rate had the 15,021 patients received traditional fall prevention interventions instead of PEVS fall prevention interventions. The overall fall rate of 1.50 falls per 1000 days of surveillance demonstrates the effectiveness of PEVS. It is especially encouraging to see that the fall rate in the oldest age group, namely, those 85 years of age and older, who are most vulnerable to injury, the fall rate was 0.38 falls per 1000 days of surveillance.

Finally, it is worth pointing out that the success of any patient care plan depends on an organization's culture, reliability of implementation, staff attitude, and fidelity to capturing accurate and meaningful data on effectiveness and efficiency.

MORE RESEARCH NEEDED

More research is needed on PEVS engagement activities, such as verbal interventions and alarm rates, and their impact on outcomes as well as patient selection. This study is the first to capture elopement from room and create a rate for observed line, tube, or drain dislodgement. With constant patient observation as implemented in PEVS, organizations can better document the true scope or adverse events occurring during patients' hospitalization. More research is needed to understand patient selection for adverse events that occur in patient rooms, including but not limited to self-harm attempts and violence against caregivers. With the vast opportunity in this field, it will be exciting to see future research outcomes.

An important piece of our findings is that in just 1 year of measuring patients on PEVS, for an average length of stay of less 3 days of surveillance, the fall rate and the rate of fall reduction with PEVS far exceeds the aggregate fall and fall rate reduction among all of the hospitals enrolled in Centers for Medicare & Medicaid Services Hospital Engagement Network/Hospital Innovation Improvement Networks (2010–2014).

The data from our study show the rapid contribution of PEVS technology on patient safety. The incidence of falls, room elopement, and line, tube, or drain dislodgement that happened for patients selected for PEVS were rare. The safety net provided by PEVS is so expansive that the many additional prevented adverse events reported through this program are beyond the scope of this article. PEVS allows monitoring staff to see and correct unsafe environments by alerting nursing staff, redirecting patients to stay in bed because a nurse is on the way to help, observing respiratory distress, recognizing the signs of delirium, and much more. With the data observed and reported through implementing PEVS technology, organizations are best positioned to correct root causes of harm and create a real-time, broad safety net for patients.

REFERENCES

1. James J. A new, evidence-based estimate of patient harms associated with hospital care. J Patient Saf 2013;9:122–8.
2. Levant S, Chari K, DeFrances CJ. Hospitalizations for patients age 85 and over in the United States, 2000-2010. NCHS Data Brief 2015;182:1–8.
3. Agency for Healthcare Research and Quality. Declines in hospital-acquired conditions from 2014 to 2016 2018. Available at: http://www.ahrq.gov/research/data/data-infographics/images/hac-rates-decline.html. Accessed July 31, 2018.
4. Agency for Healthcare Research and Quality. AHRQ National Scorecard on hospital-acquired conditions updated baseline rates and preliminary results 2014–2016. Available at: https://www.ahrq.gov/sites/default/files/wysiwyg/professionals/quality-patient-safety/pfp/natlhacratereport-rebaselining2014-2016_0.pdf. Accessed July 31, 2018.
5. Inouye SK, Brown CJ, Tinett ME. Medicare nonpayment, hospital falls, and unintended consequences. N Engl J Med 2009;360:2390–3.
6. Oliver D, Healey F, Haines T. Preventing falls and fall-related injuries in hospitals. Clin Geriatr Med 2010;26(4):645–95.
7. The Joint Commission. Sentinel alert data. General information. Quarter 2 update. Available at: https://www.jointcommission.org/assets/1/18/General_Information_2Q_2017.pdf. Accessed July 31, 2018.
8. Mitchell MD, Lavenbeg JG, Trotta R, et al. Hourly rounding to improve nursing responsiveness: a systematic review. J Nurs Adm 2014;44(9):462–72.
9. Tzeng HM, Titler MG, Ronis DL, et al. The contribution of staff call light response time to fall and injurious fall rates: an exploratory study in four US hospitals using archived hospital data. BMC Health Serv Res 2012;12:84.
10. Shever LL, Titler MG, Lehan Mackin M, et al. Fall prevention practices in adult medical-surgical nursing units described by nurse managers. West J Nurs Res 2010;33(3):385–97.

11. Tideiksaar R, Feiner CF, Maby J. Falls prevention: the efficacy of a non-intrusive falls monitor in an acute care setting. Mt Sinai J Med 1993;60(6):522–7.
12. Sahota O. Vitamin D and inpatient falls. Age Ageing 2009;38(3):339–40.
13. Shorr RI, Chandler AM, Mion LC, et al. Effects of an intervention to increase bed alarm use to prevent falls in hospitalized patients. A cluster randomized trial. Ann Intern Med 2012;157(10):692–9.
14. Jeffers S, Searcey P, Boyle K, et al. Centralized video monitoring for patient safety: a Denver Health lean journey. Nurs Econ 2013;31(6):298–306.
15. Burtson PL, Vento L. Sitter reduction through mobile monitoring. A nurse driven sitter protocol and administrative oversight. J Nurs Adm 2015;45(7–8):363–9.
16. Votruba L, Graham B, Sayed A, et al. Video monitoring to reduce falls and patient companion costs. Nurs Econ 2016;34(4):185–9.
17. Westle MB, Burkert GR, Paulus RA. Reducing inpatient falls by integrating new technology with workflow redesign. Case study. NEJM Catalyst. Available at: https://catalyst.nejm.org/reducing-inpatient-falls-virtual-sitter. Accessed July 31, 2018.
18. Cournan M, Fusco-Gessick B, Wright L. Improving patient safety through video monitoring. Rehabil Nurs 2018;43(2):111–5.
19. Methods For De-identification Of Phi, HHS Office of the Secretary, Office for Civil Rights- OCR - Available at: https://www.hhs.gov/hipaa/for-professionals/privacy/special-topics/de-identification/index.html. Accessed August 3, 2018.
20. Jones CJ, Rikli RE, Beam W. A 30-s chair stand test as a measure of lower body strength in community-residing older adults. Res Q Exerc Sport 1999;70(2):113–9.

Redesigning a Fall Prevention Program in Acute Care: Building on Evidence

Viktoriya Fridman, DNP, RN, ANP-BC*

KEYWORDS

- Fall prevention • Purposeful rounding • Toileting • Patient safety

KEY POINTS

- In-hospital falls are a critical clinical and legal problem.
- Implementation of an appropriate evidence-based fall reduction program can reduce inpatient falls.
- The practice of fall prevention in acute care settings should be shifted from hourly rounding to purposeful rounding as part of the culture change in acute care health care organizations.
- The hallmark of purposeful rounding is to meet the patient's essentials around comfort, safety, and toileting needs.

INTRODUCTION

In-hospital falls are a critical clinical and legal problem. However, there is a lack of concrete evidence on effective fall reduction programs in acute care facilities. Through the implementation of an appropriate evidence-based fall reduction program, patient outcomes can be significantly improved while decreasing the costs associated with complications of falls. Evidence-based fall prevention initiatives are consistent with a multistep broad approach and require effective leadership and innovation. Current practices need to be redesigned to ensure that the fall prevention initiatives in the acute care setting are optimized, consistent, and transformational. The purpose of this project was to explore the gap between fall prevention practice in acute care settings that is formed around hourly rounding activity as a meaningful task and a practice that is a driving force to decrease patient falls and injuries in acute care medical patients.

Disclosure: The author has nothing to disclose.
Hunter-Bellevue School of Nursing, New York, NY, USA
* 425 E 25th St, New York, NY, 10010.
E-mail address: viktoriya.fridman@hunter.cuny.edu

Clin Geriatr Med 35 (2019) 265–271
https://doi.org/10.1016/j.cger.2019.01.006
geriatric.theclinics.com

The fall prevention program in a large community teaching hospital was designated with the goal to improve patient outcomes and organizational performance by changing the organizational culture around fall safety, thus decreasing total patient falls and patient injury falls per 1000 patient days. The importance of falls in acute care settings and the need for current restructuring practices were a part of an organizational transformation. According to the National Database of Nursing Quality Indicators (NDNQI) definition of a patient fall, it is a sudden, unintentional descent, with or without injury to the patient, that results in the patient coming to rest on the floor, on or against some other surface (eg, a counter), on another person, or on an object (eg, a trash can).[1] Inpatient falls result in adverse patient outcomes, morbidity, and an increase in health care costs.[2] Falls of hospitalized vulnerable adults can be severe and have potentially life-threatening consequences for patients. Each year, somewhere between 700,000 and 1,000,000 people in the United States fall in the hospital.[3] Of those who fall, 20% to 30% suffer moderate to severe injuries that impair mobility and increase the risk of early death.[3] US hospitals demonstrated that 38% to 47% of falls were associated with toilet-related activities that occurred in the bathrooms.[4] According to the US Centers for Disease Control and Prevention, one-third of Americans aged 65 and older fall each year.[3]

IDENTIFICATION OF NEED

The significance and prevalence of falls have been identified as an immediate need for change. According to the Joint Commission alerts for health care facilities, falls with serious injury are consistently among the top 10 reported sentinel events.[5] Also, each year, nationally, about 700,000 to 1,000,000 people fall in the hospital.[6] The prevalence of falls in acute hospitals ranges between 3.3 and 11.5 falls per 1000 patient days.[6] Nearly 25% of falls in a hospital result in patient injury. Past research has highlighted numerous modifiable risk factors that have contributed to patient falls, including various geriatric syndromes, gait disorders, and specific classes of medications. Hospitalized patients have a higher chance of immobility and thus are considered high-risk. Being bed-confined is a part of the hospitalization process and may increase the likelihood that an already vulnerable patient population will experience additional deterioration in cognitive and physical performance.[6] This can result in an inability to perform basic activities of daily living. Toileting needs are the highest identified risk factor, occurring in approximately 40% of all hospital falls.[4] Much of the data on the causes show that falls can be the direct result of patients receiving Ambien. Based on a retrospective cohort study on zolpidem, this medication was identified as an independent risk factor for inpatient falls.[7] Zolpidem was reported to decrease balance and was often associated with inpatient falls, even though it is a common hypnotic medication used in a hospital setting. Health care providers have to understand and be aware that zolpidem use in patients is a critical and modifiable risk factor for falls.[7] The impairment of cognitive abilities that is commonly associated with delirium is among the risk factors that contribute to the rates of patient falls during hospitalization in the geriatric patient population. The critical features of delirium include acute confusion state, decline in attention span, and disorganized thinking that affects the safe mobility and patient compliance with various fall prevention protocols. According to a recent study, 96% of the hospitalized geriatric patients had a documented condition of delirium in their charts.[8] The condition of cognitive impairment increases the frequency of patient falls and injuries due to falls. Additionally, the clinical associations of patients receiving Ambien with delirium presence are challenging to this point of view. Integration of early delirium recognition and management of patient-specific risk factors, such as cognitive impairment, in a fall prevention program in acute care settings is highly recommended by literature.[9]

To combat inpatient falls, rounding has become the selected process in which individuals are intentionally checking on patients at regular intervals to target individual risk elements and meet their needs proactively.[10] Nurses can increase patient safety and reduce patient falls in the hospital setting through hourly rounding with the incorporation of prevention, identification, and proper management with the focus of prevention, detection, and management of adjustable falls risk factors. The main parts of hourly rounds include decreasing anxiety by using keywords and addressing pain, toileting, position, and possessions, in addition to evaluating the environment for safety concerns, telling the patient when the nursing staff will come back to check on the patient, and focusing on delirium detection and management. In this article, the definition of toileting includes all activities related to elimination needs, which include but are not limited to getting out of bed, ambulating from the bed to the bathroom, using the toilet, ambulating from the bathroom back to the bed, and getting back into the bed. Toileting-related falls should be given serious consideration during patient assessment and hourly rounding.

When implementing traditional hourly rounding, the team noted the signatures of the nursing staff in the hourly rounding logs. Does it happen every hour? To answer the question, the team conducted staff evaluations of randomly chosen patient units. The typical nurse response to the question was, "We are always in the room!" Are they in the room for the purpose of rounding or performing various nursing tasks not associated with the patient needs? The most commonly observed scenario was that the staff approached hourly rounding needs by asking the patient, "Are you okay?" This lacked the attention to the personal needs. The gap analysis in practice uncovered that patient falls associated with toileting needs occurred, on average, 15 minutes following nurse hourly rounding check on the patient. The journey in the large teaching hospital to reduce falls and injuries began with the creation of a Fall Prevention Committee in 2012. The initiation phase consisted of creating a core team that included a frontline nurse, frontline leadership, and senior leadership for commitment and support. The organizational data analysis identified that more than 40% of all falls occurred while patients were trying to get to the toilet, return from the toilet, or while attempting to exit the bed to get to the toilet. It became evident that the existing program did not ensure a nurse-driven patient-centered team approach to fall prevention. Furthermore, hourly rounding evaluation at the unit level revealed gaps in staff knowledge. These factors suggested a need to redesign the existing fall prevention program by adopting best practices with specific nursing interventions to minimize the risk of falling. On evaluating the fall prevention program, the following goals were identified:

- Improve patient outcomes and organizational performance
- Decrease hospital total patient falls per 1000 patient days
- Decrease hospital total patient injury falls per 1000 patient days
- Change organizational culture around fall safety
- Decrease severity of injuries from falls
- Decrease incidence of falls related to toileting.

Fig. 1 demonstrates the following core changes to practice were proposed and implemented:

- Evidence-based fall prevention assessment tool aligned with the target interventions
- Standardized provider assessment via electronic medical record

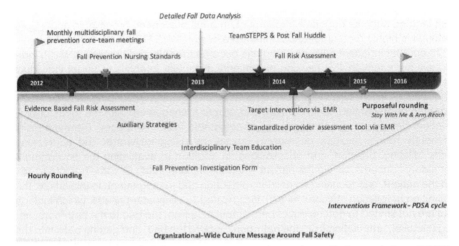

Fig. 1. Redesigning fall prevention program. EMR, electronic medical record; TeamSTEPPS, Team Strategies and Tools to Enhance Performance and Patient Safety.

- Purposeful rounding around toileting
- Developed the Stay With Me/Arm Reach program.

METHODS

The cycle consists of 4 steps: plan, do, study, and act (PDSA). It allows the organization and its employees to accept the changes that are taking place in the organization. In the planning step, it is imperative to define the problem, identify all the parties that need to be involved, come up with a plan, and form a prediction. The next step is to roll out the project and then review the effectiveness of the project over a period of time. The following step is to analyze the data to make predictions about the possible solution to the problem at hand. In the last phase of the PDSA cycle, a decision on whether or not to implement changes permanently is made, with follow-up and monitoring. The primary method to change the culture of care delivery is to change reactive to proactive behavior. It is imperative for nursing staff to understand that being in the room and asking, "Are you okay?" does not qualify as rounding. The behaviors of purposeful rounding give patients a framework to express their needs and convey the nurse's concern for the patient's well-being.[10]

Safe toileting procedures are based on anchoring purposeful rounding behaviors, embedding a targeted toileting schedule, and implementing the Stay With Me/Arm Reach policy. The nursing staff should state to the patient, "Let me take you to the bathroom," instead of asking the patient, "Would you like to use the bathroom?"

PDSA cycles **(Fig. 2)** were used to implement and anchor changes to the fall prevention program. One cycle used the simulation laboratory to observe previous practice of hourly rounding. After going through the initial simulation session, the participant and facilitator debriefed to review the difference between hourly rounding and purposeful rounding, as well as the expected behaviors. **Table 1** reveals that the previous practice of hourly rounding did not ensure that the core patient needs associated with rounding were adequately addressed. After debriefing, all participants (nurses and patient care technicians [PCTs]) were able to develop the language and dialog to address care behaviors with purposeful rounding.

The purpose of this observational study was to describe the effectiveness of a nursing quality improvement activity for a fall prevention program, with a particular

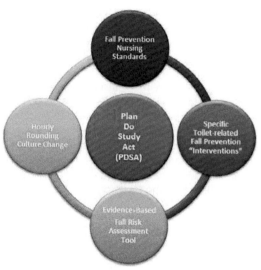

Fig. 2. PDSA cycles.

focus on specific evidence-based nursing interventions to minimize the risk of the patient falls. To achieve a practice change, the team recognized the need for a so-called change champion team that included of a group of individuals with interest in fall prevention to disseminate the culture change across the organization. The team consisted of frontline nursing and leadership team representatives. The goal of this team was to explore and adopt innovative practices that could result in a decrease in falls. A clear vision of fall prevention awareness, including capacity, capability, and sustainability, was established.

IMPLEMENTATION

A stepwise approach to decreasing inpatient falls and falls due to toileting was proposed. The pilot study revealed that only 13.3% of participants, including registered nurses (RN) and patient care technicians (PCTs) (see **Table 1**) addressed patients about their toileting needs. Often, nurses or PCTs reacted to the problem by saying, "Let me see if you are dry or clean," instead of proactively preventing the problem

Table 1	
Hourly rounding behaviors	
Behavior Validation	**Knowledge Before Debriefing**
Explain the purpose of hourly rounding at initial visit	13.3%
Describe purposeful rounding schedule	26.7%
Pain	53.3%
Position	73.3%
Potty	13.3%
Possessions	73.3%
Communicate when you will return	33.3%
Is there anything else that I can do for you?	46.7%

by saying, "It is time for you to use the bathroom, let me assist you." This statement works best for patients with cognitive impairment. With the patient experience paramount, the goal is the reduction in fall-related patient harm while anchoring purposeful rounding behaviors, embedding a targeted toileting schedule, and implementing the Stay With Me/Arm Reach guideline. The rollout of the restructured fall prevention initiative began as a pilot program on a medical unit where the process was readily embraced by geriatric resource nurse champions. Through education, frontline nurse involvement, and redesigning fall prevention approach, hourly rounding was promoted as a proactive falls prevention strategy with the goal of decreasing falls and promoting patient safety, health, and comfort. This study presented an opportunity to hardwire the culture around purposeful rounding as a standard of care across the organization. **Box 1** itemizes specific strategies that acute care organizations may consider in the redesigning of hourly rounding with the focus on falls prevention.

RESULTS

The overall fall prevention program evaluation was based on the NDNQI falls per 1000 patient days (**Fig. 3**). A process change on a pilot medical unit was effectively implemented. At the start of educational and simulation sessions for purposeful rounding, a decrease in patient falls, injuries related to falls, and incidence of falls linked to toileting became evident. This decline was likely not entirely related to the revised rounding practice and testing of the Stay With Me/Arm Reach on the pilot unit. Key program elements, such as integrating the evidence-based fall risk model and assessment-related interventions, were all part of the process change in the acute care setting.

Results of this performance improvement initiative show that direct care nursing staff making purposeful point-of-care rounds will experience positive outcomes in preventing patient falls. Preventing patient falls is certainly not new to nursing. Instead, this is falls prevention with a fresh twist on structuring fall risk factors along with target intervention by engaging the frontline nursing team in providing high-quality patient care. A clear relationship has been established between the diagnosis of delirium, the patient's toileting needs, high-risk prescription medication, ambulation impairment, and an increase in the number of patient falls. It is imperative to promote various prevention, detection, and proper management aspects of evidence-based programs that are designed to improve the outcomes of patient care and decrease the fall rates in various acute care facilities. Results suggest that fall prevention is complicated, and careful planning, implementation, and evaluation are required for successful nursing practice change. Health care providers must possess proper knowledge of modifiable risk factors to improve care plans and reach the overall objective of providing safe patient care.[8]

Box 1
Purposeful rounding implementation strategies

- Establish behaviors of purposeful rounding
- Evaluate RN and PCT baseline knowledge and identify gaps through simulation sessions
- Provide education and fill gaps through debriefing session after initial simulation
- Observe changes in behavior during simulation
- Identify needs for further education through teach-back methodology
- Performance validation

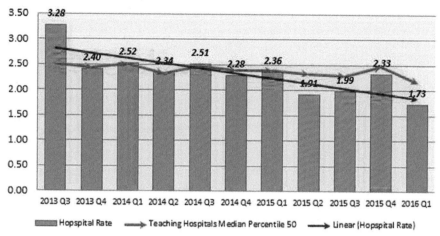

Fig. 3. Hospital total falls rate per 1000 patient days.

These findings indicate that all frontline nursing staff should be appropriately educated and trained in proactive fall prevention initiatives to anticipate hospitalized adult needs. Team engagement and staff buy-in are critical to successful implementation and compliance with the policy. Empowering the nursing team through the use of a patient-centered approach and clinical judgment, instead of requesting their performance to be similar to preprogrammed methods, was part of a transformational design of this evidence-based fall prevention program in an acute care setting.

REFERENCES

1. Staggs VS, Davidson J, Dunton N, et al. Challenges in defining and categorizing falls on diverse unit types. J Nurs Care Qual 2015;30(2):106–12.
2. Rheaume J, Fruh S. Retrospective case reviews of adult inpatient falls in the acute care setting. Medsurg Nurs 2015;24(5):318–24.
3. CDC - Older adult falls - falls among older adults: an overview - home and recreational safety - injury center. Available at: http://www.cdc.gov/homeandrecreationalsafety/falls/adultfalls.html. Accessed February 10, 2017.
4. Tzeng H. Understanding the prevalence of inpatient falls associated with toileting in adult acute care settings. J Nurs Care Qual 2010;25(1):22–30.
5. Joint Commission. Preventing falls and fall-related injuries in health care facilities. Sentinel Event Alert 2015;(55):1.
6. Ganz DA, Huang C, Saliba D, et al. Preventing falls in hospitals: a toolkit for improving quality of care. Ann Intern Med 2013;158(5 Pt 2):390–6.
7. Kolla BP. Zolpidem is independently associated with increased risk of inpatient falls. J Hosp Med 2012;8(1):1–6.
8. Lakatos BE, Capasso V, Mitchell MT, et al. Falls in the general hospital: association with delirium, advanced age, and specific surgical procedures. Psychosomatics 2009;50(3):218–26.
9. Ambrose AF, Paul G, Hausdorff JM. Risk factors for falls among older adults: a review of the literature. Maturitas 2013;75(1):51–61.
10. Mitchell MD, Lavenberg JG, Trotta RL, et al. Hourly rounding to improve nursing responsiveness. JONA: The Journal of Nursing Administration 2014;44(9):462–72.

Preventing Falls in Hospitalized Patients
State of the Science

Jennifer H. LeLaurin, MPH[a], Ronald I. Shorr, MD, MS[b],*

KEYWORDS

- Accidental falls • Hospitals • Prevention • Aged • Alarms • Restraints • Nursing

KEY POINTS

- Falls in hospitalized patients result in significant burdens to patients and medical organizations.
- Despite the multiplicity of "positive" quality assurance demonstrations of fall prevention interventions, these studies should not be viewed as "evidence" of effectiveness.
- Few controlled interventions exceed usual care in preventing hospital falls when tested rigorously.
- There is a pressing need for large, well-designed trials of hospital fall prevention interventions.

INTRODUCTION

Although hospital falls have been decreasing over the past several years, they remain a significant problem.[1] Patient falls are the most common adverse events reported in hospitals.[2–5] Each year, roughly 700,000 to 1 million patient falls occur in United States hospitals, resulting in around 250,000 injuries and up to 11,000 deaths.[6] About 2% of hospitalized patients fall at least once during their stay.[7,8] Approximately 1 in 4 falls results in injury, with about 10% resulting in serious injury.[9]

Inpatient falls result in significant physical and economic burdens to patients (increased injury and mortality rates and decreased quality of life) as well as to medical organizations (increased lengths of stay, medical care costs, and litigation).[10,11] In 2008, the Centers for Medicare and Medicaid Services (CMS) stopped reimbursing

Disclosures: Dr R.I. Shorr serves as an expert witness in hospital falls cases.
[a] Center of Innovation on Disability and Rehabilitation Research (CINDRR), Malcom Randall VA Medical Center, 1601 SW Archer Road, CINDRR (151B), Gainesville, FL 32608, USA; [b] Geriatric Research Education and Clinical Center (GRECC), University of Florida, Malcom Randall VA Medical Center, 1601 SW Archer Road, GRECC (182), Gainesville, FL 32608, USA
* Corresponding author.
E-mail address: Rshorr@ufl.edu

hospitals for fall-related injuries.[12] Given significant financial pressure, hospitals are seeking a "silver bullet" for fall prevention.[13]

Hospitals use various "guidelines" for fall prevention.[14–16] In general these include (1) identify patients who are at high risk of falling and (2) use clinical judgment to decide which of a multitude of fall prevention strategies to use to reduce fall risk. Not surprisingly, there is considerable heterogeneity among the guidelines, which adds to confusion on the "correct approach" to fall prevention; this is promoting the uptake of time- and labor-intensive approaches to fall prevention into "standard of care."[17] The lack of clarity of prevention guidelines may add to the cognitive burden of patient care and potentially increases patient risk.[18–20]

Although there is a growing body of research on fall prevention in the community-dwelling elderly, findings from these studies are not necessarily generalizable to the hospital environment.[17] Hospital patients have a myriad of acute and chronic illnesses that limit judgment and mobility, and they must navigate a new and unfamiliar environment. Furthermore, staffing and even unit design considerations may play into fall risk. Short lengths of stay offer a brief window of time to conduct interventions, rendering some strategies (eg, exercise programs) impractical. The unique organizational culture and leadership structures of hospitals require specific implementation strategies. Thus, it is imperative to examine fall prevention intervention strategies specific to the hospital setting.

STUDY DESIGNS

Although this article is by no means a complete review of study designs, its goal is to familiarize the reader with the strengths and limitations of the types of research often used to test fall prevention interventions.

Quality Improvement Studies

Many studies on fall prevention in hospitals take the form of a quality improvement (QI) study. The goal of QI studies is *not* to generate generalizable knowledge but to share the results of a programmatic change on health outcome such as falls.[21] Many QI studies use an uncontrolled before-and-after design conducted on single nursing unit (or group of units).

There are several reasons why most QI studies should not be viewed as "evidence" of effectiveness of a fall prevention strategy. First, these studies are generally less rigorous than research studies. Pronovost and Wachter[22] state that QI studies "commonly lack clarity regarding the study population, interventions and co-interventions, outcome measurement and definitions...and what data are available may be poor in quality." QI interventions frequently contain multiple components, often not well described, which can change throughout the study. In addition, many of these interventions are led by a "champion," and it is difficult to know how much the intervention depended on the "champion." Also, without a control group it is difficult to distinguish the effect of intervention from underlying secular trends in falls. Finally, the incentive to publish a negative QI study is low, so the possibility of publication bias is high. This may explain why Hempel and colleagues[23] found that the intervention effect for fall prevention across historical control studies (often QI) was 0.77 (95% confidence interval = 0.5 to 1.18), whereas the intervention effect for fall prevention in studies with concurrent controls (often research) was 0.92 (95% confidence interval = 0.65 to 1.30).

In sum, we view QI studies as analogous to "case reports." These studies are important for hypothesis generation but do not serve as "evidence" that a fall prevention strategy is effective outside of the context of the QI initiative.

Research: Randomized Studies

Controlled trials represent a much stronger study design. Randomization and outcome assessment can occur at the patient level or at a larger level—often the nursing unit. Such designs are referred to as cluster randomized controlled trials (cRCTs). Traditionally cRCTs were conducted using a parallel design, meaning that once randomized, study units maintain intervention and control conditions throughout the duration of the study. A stepped wedge is a newer design whereby all units in the study transition from control to experimental conditions at regular intervals, called "steps," which controls for underlying secular trends.[24] This type of design is particularly advantageous when evaluating a clinical or policy strategy that has been "made" but can be rolled out at flexible dates.

There are several advantages in using a cRCT rather than a patient-randomized study for hospital fall prevention. First, the possibility of contamination of the intervention onto control patients is lessened when conducted by geographically separated staff. Second, although an intervention may be effective at the patient level (eg, none of the patients fell who had the intervention), the total number of falls a unit experiences may remain unchanged because the intervention was not applied to the "appropriate" patients or so much attention was paid to the intervention patients on the unit that "different" patients fell. Thus, an intervention could be efficacious for individual patients but not effective in practice.

In a cRCT, units should be followed for several months before randomization to establish baseline rates, then randomized to intervention and control conditions using methods that would ensure that baseline fall rates are similar between intervention and control units. Follow-up should be long enough to minimize the study novelty and to allow units to establish stable fall rates. To minimize ascertainment bias it is important that the visibility of the study remain approximately equal between intervention and control units. To address secular trends in fall rates, the effect of the intervention should be tested using the interaction of the slope of the rate of falls in the unit type (intervention or control) and the time (before and after initiation of the intervention).

Research: Nonrandomized Studies

Although RCTs yield the highest level of evidence, some universally applied interventions (eg, national policy changes) cannot be studied in a controlled manor.[25] In such cases, useful evidence can be derived from large, credible parallel or before-and-after studies in which the effect size cannot easily be attributable to confounders, and where efforts have been made to control for secular trends.[26]

SINGLE FALL PREVENTION INTERVENTIONS
Fall Risk Identification

The use of fall risk prediction tools is widespread, but their value in hospital fall prevention interventions is questionable.[27–29] First, it is important distinguish between fall risk assessments and fall prediction or screening tools. Risk assessments usually consist of a checklist of risk factors for falls, but do not provide a score or value for the patient's fall risk. Predictive tools use these known risk factors to calculate a score for the patient's risk of falling, with established cutoffs to identify risk level.

Some tools have demonstrated acceptable sensitivity and specificity in single studies, but the reported predictive values of these tools vary by study design, setting, and population.[27,28,30] Furthermore, a patient's risk for falling is transitory, requiring periodic reassessment. Few tools have been validated with specifically older hospital patients in mind, and a recent systematic review concluded that existing tools do not have sufficient specificity and sensitivity to be effectively used in this population.[31]

The lack of evidence supporting the use of predictive tools led to 2013 National Institute for Health and Care Excellence guidelines, which explicitly recommended *against* the routine use of fall prediction tools, instead advising that all inpatients older than 65 years be considered at high risk.[32] The Agency for Healthcare Research and Quality (AHRQ) cautions that it is more important to identify and address a patient's specific fall risk factors than to determine their risk for falling.[3] Despite this, fall risk screening tools are frequently used to identify patients for intervention,[23] often relying on "home-made" tools without established psychometric properties.[4] Although these tools have the potential to tailor fall prevention strategies to specific patient risk factors,[33] they predict falls no better than nursing judgment.[34]

Alarms

Alarm systems are designed to reduce falls by alerting staff when patients attempt to leave a bed or chair without assistance. They can also function as a reminder to patients to call for assistance before getting up. There are several types of alarm systems in use, including pressure mats, infrared movement detectors, cord-activated alarms, and wearable devices.[35] Alarms are disruptive and may be especially disturbing to cognitively impaired patients, contributing to confusion and agitation; they also restrict mobility and independence. In United States nursing homes alarms are considered a type of restraint, and facilities can be penalized for indiscriminate use of the devices.[36]

There is now strong evidence that alarms are ineffective as a fall prevention maneuver in hospitals.[37,38] A large cRCT tested the effectiveness of bed/chair alarm systems to prevent falls in 16 general medical, surgical, and specialty units in a United States community hospital.[37] Although the intervention successfully increased alarm use, there was no significant effect on falls or use of physical restraint. In an RCT performed in 3 acute wards in a United Kingdom hospital, Sahota and colleagues[38] found that alarms did not reduce fall rates and were not cost effective. The AHRQ has cautioned that there is an overreliance on alarms as a fall prevention measure,[3] yet alarms remain in use by more than 90% of nurse managers.[39]

There are a few possible explanations for the ineffectiveness of alarms as a fall prevention strategy. Reliance on alarms assumes that staff have enough time to intervene before a fall, which could be only a matter of seconds. Alarms may decrease vigilance by giving staff a false sense of security. Finally, The Joint Commission has expressed concerns about excessive hospital noise leading to general "alarm fatigue."[40]

Although the current body of evidence does not support the effectiveness of alarms as a fall prevention measure in hospitals, there is promising new technology that may better predict and prevent falls.[41,42] These new systems and devices have the potential to serve as effective and sustainable fall prevention strategies.

Sitters

Sitters, also known as companions or "specials," are a potentially effective yet costly fall prevention strategy. Sitters provide 1-to-1 surveillance for patients deemed at high risk for falls and may additionally provide therapeutic care. Guidelines for the use of sitters and their duties, qualifications, and training vary among hospitals.[43,44]

There is indirect evidence of sitter effectiveness, but no RCTs of sitters as a single intervention have been performed to date. The evidence supporting effectiveness of sitters has been limited to small observational studies conducted in a single hospital—each with its own definition of what constitutes a sitter.[45–48] In addition to the limited evidence of effectiveness, there is the possibility that sitters may have an adverse effect on patient care; for example, to save on costs existing staff may be employed as sitters, potentially placing other patients at risk. Despite the lack of evidence, sitters are recommended in numerous fall prevention guidelines.[49]

Sitters represent a considerable expense, with annual costs of over $1 million reported.[45,50] These costs are rising and are typically not reimbursable by third-party payers.[45,51] Owing to their expense, hospitals are increasingly interested in reducing sitter use without negatively affecting patient safety. Several initiatives have successfully reduced sitter use without increasing fall rates.[43,52]

In sum, patient sitters are costly and hospitals discourage their use. Although not studied rigorously, whether sitters prevent falls is not well established.[43] Feil and Wallace[49] found that more than 4 of 5 falls that occurred with a sitter present were unassisted, reinforcing the hypothesis that sitters are not a panacea for hospital falls.

Intentional Rounding

In an effort to increase patient satisfaction and reduce patient harm, many hospitals have instituted intentional rounding. Rounding is a proactive approach to meeting patient needs that involves bedside checks at regular intervals, usually every 1 to 2 hours. The quality of evidence for rounding is weak, with most of the literature consisting of QI studies.[53,54] Difficulties with adherence and sustainability of rounding initiatives are widely reported,[55–57] and introduction of the practice is often perceived as a top-down approach that restricts staff autonomy.[57] Other barriers include increased workload, competing priorities, poor documentation, inadequate education, and lack of staff buy-in.[55,56] Thus, even if stronger evidence supporting the effectiveness of rounding is produced, the feasibility of the strategy as a sustainable fall prevention practice is uncertain.

Patient Education

There is some evidence that education is an effective component of multifactorial interventions,[58] but the body of evidence on their effectiveness as a single intervention is limited. Haines and colleagues[58] performed an RCT of a multimedia education intervention combined with 1-on-1 follow-up from a health professional. Although the intervention did not significantly reduce fall-related outcomes overall, subgroup analysis of cognitively intact patients who received the intervention showed a 50% reduction in fall rates. When the same intervention was tested in a cRCT in 8 hospital rehabilitation wards, there was a significant reduction in rates of falls and falls resulting in injury.[59] These results may be explained by the fact that patients in rehabilitation wards tend to be more cognitively intact than those in acute settings. Thus, although patient education is potentially effective in reducing hospital falls for certain patients, it is not suitable for patients with cognitive impairment, a common risk factor for inpatient falls.[60]

Environmental Modifications

The physical environment can be an important contributor to falls. Of a total of 538 hospital falls resulting in death or permanent loss of function that were reviewed by The Joint Commission, 209 (39%) identified the physical environment as part of the root cause.[8] Small studies have explored the impact of a variety of environmental modifications. One RCT found that fewer falls occurred on vinyl flooring compared with carpet, but the findings were limited by a small sample size and low fall rate during the 9-month trial.[61] A cRCT found no evidence that low-low beds reduced rates of falls or injuries from falls.[62] Other interventions have included visual cues (eg, signage, wristbands), lighting, and the use of special rooms for high-risk patients.[63–65] Some of these fall prevention efforts have resulted in patient harm; for example, in 2005 the Food and Drug Administration issued a recall of enclosed beds after reports of patient injury and death from entrapment.[66]

Physical Restraints

There is considerable controversy surrounding the use of physical restraints in hospital settings.[5,67] Patients who require restraints suffer a loss of dignity and autonomy; furthermore, restraints may also cause agitation, delirium, pressure ulcers, deconditioning, strangulation, and death.[68,69] Data suggest that restraints may not protect, but actually increase the risk of falling or sustaining an injurious fall.[70–72]

Unfortunately, on the part of both health professionals and patients, there is a perception that restraints reduce the risk of falling, and they are often used as a "last resort" to protect patients from falling.[67,73,74] This perception of effective physical restraint as a strategy to prevent falls has persisted despite the increasingly restrictive regulations and standards from the CMS and The Joint Commission limiting its use.[75,76]

Nonslip Socks

Nonslip socks are often provided to hospitalized patients under the assumption that they will provide additional traction to prevent falls. In contrast to manufacturers' claims, research has cast doubt on the slip-resistant properties of these products.[77] The small body of research on nonslip socks has not provided evidence of their efficacy as a fall prevention strategy.[78] Furthermore, nonslip socks carry the risk of spreading drug-resistant infection in hospitals.[79] Given the lack of evidence of effectiveness and potential to spread infection, a patient's own footwear remains the safest option for fall prevention.

MULTIFACTORIAL INTERVENTIONS

Given the multitude of factors contributing to falls, it is intuitive that multicomponent interventions would be most effective in improving fall outcomes. Although fall prevention guidelines typically recommend the use of multicomponent interventions,[3,14,16,32] there have been few controlled trials of multicomponent interventions. Of these, some have found a reduction in fall rates[80,81] whereas others have reported no intervention effect.[82,83] Barker and colleagues[83] recently conducted the largest cRCT of a hospital fall prevention intervention to date in 24 wards in 6 Australian hospitals (n = 46,245 admissions). Despite successful implementation of the 6-PACK program, the intervention did not produce lower rates of falls or fall-related injuries.

The limited number of high-quality studies and heterogeneity among intervention sites make it challenging to combine studies for quantitative overviews. In a 2012 Cochrane review,[84] pooled analysis of 4 small multicomponent RCTs revealed an overall reduction in fall rate ratio (0.69, 95% confidence interval 0.49 to 0.96) but not injurious falls. However, 3 of the cited studies included subacute care units and the fourth was conducted in a single geriatric orthopedic unit. A 2012 meta-analysis of 6 acute care interventions[85] found a statistically significant but small reduction in fall rates (odds ratio 0.9, 95% confidence interval 0.83 to 0.99). A 2013 updated review[2] supported the evidence for multicomponent interventions, additionally identifying factors associated with successful. It should be noted that none of these analyses included the most recent negative results of the 6-PACK trial; this information will be included in a forthcoming Cochrane review.

The current body of evidence on multifactorial interventions is limited in several respects. The heterogeneity of components, delivery characteristics, and target populations make it difficult to identify which specific components are effective. Implementation is a key component of any successful patient safety initiative, but there is a lack of reporting on how interventions were implemented in published studies.[23] Finally, the body of evidence also tends to be limited to older populations with a longer length of stay.[5]

SUMMARY

Although decreasing, hospital falls are a significant patient safety problem. Although there is a growing body of literature on strategies to prevent these events, most reports are uncontrolled QI studies. Even though a number of successful QI programs have been described, most controlled studies of fall prevention have been "negative." Such results are typical for any "emerging science." Thus, there is an urgent need for well-designed research studies of hospital fall prevention.

ACKNOWLEDGMENTS

The author received grants from the Veterans Health Administration (1I01HX002191) and the National Institutes of Health (R56AG051799).

REFERENCES

1. He J, Dunton N, Staggs V. Unit-level time trends in inpatient fall rates of US hospitals. Med Care 2012;50:801–7.
2. Miake-Lye IM, Hempel S, Ganz DA, et al. Inpatient fall prevention programs as a patient safety strategy: a systematic review. Ann Intern Med 2013;158:390–6.
3. Ganz DA, Huang C, Saliba D, et al. Preventing falls in hospitals: a toolkit for improving quality of care (Prepared by RAND Corporation, Boston University School of Public Health, and ECRI Institute under Contract No. HHSA290201000017I TO #1.). Rockville (MD): Agency for Healthcare Research and Quality; 2013.
4. Hempel S, Newberry S, Wang Z, et al. Review of the evidence on falls prevention in hospitals: task 4, final report. Santa Monica (CA): RAND Corporation, WR-907-AHRQ2012. Available at: http://www.rand.org/pubs/working_papers/WR907. Accessed September 21, 2014.
5. Oliver D, Healey F, Haines TP. Preventing falls and fall-related injuries in hospitals. Clin Geriatr Med 2010;26:645–92.
6. Currie L. Fall and injury prevention. In: Hughes RG, editor. Patient safety and quality: an evidence-based handbook for nurses (prepared with support from the Robert Wood Johnson Foundation). AHRQ Publication no. 08-0043. Rockville (MD): Agency for Healthcare Research and Quality; 2008. p. 196–250.
7. Agostini JV, Baker DI, Bogardus ST. Prevention of falls in hospitalized and institutionalized older people. Making health care safer: a critical analysis of patient safety practices. File Inventory, evidence report/technology assessment number 43. AHRQ Publication No. 01-E058. Chapter 26. Rockville (MD): Agency for Healthcare Research and Quality; 2001. p. 281–99.
8. Morse JM. Enhancing the safety of hospitalization by reducing patient falls. Am J Infect Control 2002;30:376–80.
9. Rubenstein LZ, Josephson KR. The epidemiology of falls and syncope. Clin Geriatr Med 2002;18:141–58.
10. The Joint Commission. Sentinel event data root causes by event type 2004-2012 2012. Available at: http://www.jointcommission.org/assets/1/18/Root_Causes_Event_Type_04_4Q2012.pdf. Accessed October 8, 2014.

11. Gulwadi GB, Calkins MP. The impact of healthcare environmental design on patient falls. Concord (CA): Center for Healthcare Design; 2008.
12. Inouye SK, Brown CJ, Tinetti ME. Medicare nonpayment, hospital falls, and unintended consequences. N Engl J Med 2009;360:2390–3.
13. Goldsack J, Cunningham J, Mascioli S. Patient falls: searching for the elusive "silver bullet". Nursing 2014;44:61–2.
14. Registered Nurses' Association of Ontario. (1) Prevention of falls and fall injuries in the older adult. (2) Prevention of falls and fall injuries in the older adult 2011 supplement. National Guideline Clearinghouse; 2011. Available at: https://rnao.ca/sites/rnao-ca/files/Prevention_of_Falls_and_Fall_Injuries_in_the_Older_Adult.pdf. Accessed August 6, 2018.
15. Hartford Institute for Geriatric Nursing. Fall prevention. In: Evidence-based geriatric nursing protocols for best practice. National Guideline Clearinghouse; 2013. Available at: https://www.guidelinecentral.com/summaries/fall-prevention-in-evidence-based-geriatric-nursing-protocols-for-best-practice/. Accessed August 6, 2018.
16. Australian Commission on Safety and Quality in Health Care. Preventing falls and harm from falls in older people: best practice guidelines for Australian hospitals. Available at: https://www.safetyandquality.gov.au/wp-content/uploads/2009/01/Guidelines-HOSP.pdf. Accessed November 6, 2018.
17. Haines TP, Waldron NG. Translation of falls prevention knowledge into action in hospitals: what should be translated and how should it be done? J Safety Res 2011;42:431–42.
18. Lopez KD, Gerling GJ, Cary MP, et al. Cognitive work analysis to evaluate the problem of patient falls in an inpatient setting. J Am Med Inform Assoc 2010;17:313–21.
19. Graham KC, Cvach M. Monitor alarm fatigue: standardizing use of physiological monitors and decreasing nuisance alarms. Am J Crit Care 2010;19:28–34 [quiz: 35].
20. Lea E, Andrews S, Hill K, et al. Beyond the 'tick and flick': facilitating best practice falls prevention through an action research approach. J Clin Nurs 2012;21:1896–905.
21. Fiore LD, Lavori PW. Integrating randomized comparative effectiveness research with patient care. N Engl J Med 2016;374:2152–8.
22. Pronovost P, Wachter R. Proposed standards for quality improvement research and publication: one step forward and two steps back. Qual Saf Health Care 2006;15:152–3.
23. Hempel S, Newberry S, Wang Z, et al. Hospital fall prevention: a systematic review of implementation, components, adherence, and effectiveness. J Am Geriatr Soc 2013;61:483–94.
24. Hemming K, Haines TP, Chilton PJ, et al. The stepped wedge cluster randomised trial: rationale, design, analysis, and reporting. BMJ 2015;350:h391.
25. Waters TM, Daniels MJ, Bazzoli GJ, et al. Effect of Medicare's nonpayment for hospital-acquired conditions: lessons for future policy. JAMA Intern Med 2015;175:347–54.
26. Soumerai SB, Ceccarelli R, Koppel R. False dichotomies and health policy research designs: randomized trials are not always the answer. J Gen Intern Med 2017;32:204–9.
27. Aranda-Gallardo M, Morales-Asencio JM, Canca-Sanchez JC, et al. Instruments for assessing the risk of falls in acute hospitalized patients: a systematic review and meta-analysis. BMC Health Serv Res 2013;13:122.

28. da Costa BR, Rutjes AW, Mendy A, et al. Can falls risk prediction tools correctly identify fall-prone elderly rehabilitation inpatients? A systematic review and meta-analysis. PLoS One 2012;7:e41061.

29. Oliver D, Daly F, Martin FC, et al. Risk factors and risk assessment tools for falls in hospital in-patients: a systematic review. Age Ageing 2004;33:122–30.

30. Haines TP, Hill K, Walsh W, et al. Design-related bias in hospital fall risk screening tool predictive accuracy evaluations: systematic review and meta-analysis. J Gerontol A Biol Sci Med Sci 2007;62:664–72.

31. Matarese M, Ivziku D, Bartolozzi F, et al. Systematic review of fall risk screening tools for older patients in acute hospitals. J Adv Nurs 2015;71:1198–209.

32. National Institute for Health and Care Excellence. Assessment and prevention of falls in older people. NICE clinical guideline 161 2013. Available at: https://www.nice.org.uk/guidance/cg161/evidence/full-guideline-pdf-190033741. Accessed August 6, 2018.

33. Dykes PC, Carroll DL, Hurley A, et al. Fall prevention in acute care hospitals: a randomized trial. JAMA 2010;304:1912–8.

34. Oliver D. Falls risk-prediction tools for hospital inpatients. Time to put them to bed? Age Ageing 2008;37:248–50.

35. Wong Shee A, Phillips B, Hill K, et al. Feasibility, acceptability, and effectiveness of an electronic sensor bed/chair alarm in reducing falls in patients with cognitive impairment in a subacute ward. J Nurs Care Qual 2014;29:253–62.

36. Centers for Medicare & Medicaid Services. State operations manual: appendix pp - guidance to surveyors for long term care facilities (Rev. 173, 11-22-17) 2018. Available at: https://www.cms.gov/Medicare/Provider-Enrollment-and-Certification/GuidanceforLawsAndRegulations/Nursing-Homes.html. Accessed July 5, 2017.

37. Shorr RI, Chandler AM, Mion LC, et al. Effects of an intervention to increase bed alarm use to prevent falls in hospitalized patients: a cluster randomized trial. Ann Intern Med 2012;157:692–9.

38. Sahota O, Drummond A, Kendrick D, et al. REFINE (REducing Falls in In-patieNt Elderly) using bed and bedside chair pressure sensors linked to radio-pagers in acute hospital care: a randomised controlled trial. Age Ageing 2014;43:247–53.

39. Shever LL, Titler MG, Mackin ML, et al. Fall prevention practices in adult medical-surgical nursing units described by nurse managers. West J Nurs Res 2011;33:385–97.

40. The Joint Commission. Hospital national patient safety goals. Goal 6: reduce the harm associated with clinical alarm systems 2013. Available at: http://www.jointcommission.org/assets/1/6/HAP_NPSG_Chapter_2014.pdf. Accessed December 13, 2014.

41. Wolf KH, Hetzer K, zu Schwabedissen HM, et al. Development and pilot study of a bed-exit alarm based on a body-worn accelerometer. Z Gerontol Geriatr 2013;46:727–33.

42. Balaguera HU, Wise D, Ng CY, et al. Using a medical intranet of things system to prevent bed falls in an Acute Care Hospital: a pilot study. J Med Internet Res 2017;19:e150.

43. Lang CE. Do sitters prevent falls? A review of the literature. J Gerontol Nurs 2014;40:24–33 [quiz: 34–5].

44. Wood VJ, Vindrola-Padros C, Swart N, et al. One to one specialling and sitters in acute care hospitals: a scoping review. Int J Nurs Stud 2018;84:61–77.

45. Spiva L, Feiner T, Jones D, et al. An evaluation of a sitter reduction program intervention. J Nurs Care Qual 2012;27:341–5.

46. Rochefort CM, Ward L, Ritchie JA, et al. Registered nurses' job demands in relation to sitter use: nested case-control study. Nurs Res 2011;60:221–30.
47. Tzeng HM, Yin CY, Grunawalt J. Effective assessment of use of sitters by nurses in inpatient care settings. J Adv Nurs 2008;64:176–83.
48. Boswell DJ, Ramsey J, Smith MA, et al. The cost-effectiveness of a patient-sitter program in an acute care hospital: a test of the impact of sitters on the incidence of falls and patient satisfaction. Qual Manag Health Care 2001;10:10–6.
49. Feil M, Wallace SC. The use of patient sitters to reduce falls: best practices. Pennsylvania Patient Safety Advisory 2014;11:8–14.
50. Salamon L, Lennon M. Decreasing companion usage without negatively affecting patient outcomes: a performance improvement project. Medsurg Nurs 2003;12: 230–6 [quiz: 237].
51. Rausch DL, Bjorklund P. Decreasing the costs of constant observation. J Nurs Adm 2010;40:75–81.
52. Bock TJ. A solution to sitters that won't fall short. Nurs Manage 2017;48:38–44.
53. Halm MA. Hourly rounds: what does the evidence indicate? Am J Crit Care 2009; 18:581–4.
54. Mitchell MD, Lavenberg JG, Trotta RL, et al. Hourly rounding to improve nursing responsiveness: a systematic review. J Nurs Adm 2014;44:462–72.
55. Toole N, Meluskey T, Hall N. A systematic review: barriers to hourly rounding. J Nurs Manag 2016;24:283–90.
56. Deitrick LM, Baker K, Paxton H, et al. Hourly rounding: challenges with implementation of an evidence-based process. J Nurs Care Qual 2012;27:13–9.
57. Christiansen A, Coventry L, Graham R, et al. Intentional rounding in acute adult healthcare settings: a systematic mixed-method review. J Clin Nurs 2018;27: 1759–92.
58. Haines TP, Hill KD, Bennell KL, et al. Patient education to prevent falls in subacute care. Clin Rehabil 2006;20:970–9.
59. Hill AM, McPhail SM, Waldron N, et al. Fall rates in hospital rehabilitation units after individualised patient and staff education programmes: a pragmatic, stepped-wedge, cluster-randomised controlled trial. Lancet 2015;385:2592–9.
60. Evans D, Hodgkinson B, Lambert L, et al. Falls risk factors in the hospital setting: a systematic review. Int J Nurs Pract 2001;7:38–45.
61. Donald IP, Pitt K, Armstrong E, et al. Preventing falls on an elderly care rehabilitation ward. Clin Rehabil 2000;14:178–85.
62. Haines TP, Bell RA, Varghese PN. Pragmatic, cluster randomized trial of a policy to introduce low-low beds to hospital wards for the prevention of falls and fall injuries. J Am Geriatr Soc 2010;58:435–41.
63. Mills PB, Neily J, Luan D, et al. Using aggregate root cause analysis to reduce falls. Jt Comm J Qual Patient Saf 2005;31:21–31.
64. Hitcho EB, Krauss MJ, Birge S, et al. Characteristics and circumstances of falls in a hospital setting. J Gen Intern Med 2004;19:732–9.
65. Taylor E, Hignett S. The SCOPE of Hospital falls: a systematic mixed studies review. HERD 2016;9:86–109.
66. US Food and Drug Administration. Class 1 device recall Vail 1000 enclosed bed system 2005. Available at: https://www.accessdata.fda.gov/scripts/cdrh/cfdocs/cfres/res.cfm?id=39028. Accessed August 6, 2018.
67. Vassallo M, Wilkinson C, Stockdale R, et al. Attitudes to restraint for the prevention of falls in hospital. Gerontology 2005;51:66–70.
68. Miles SH, Irvine P. Deaths caused by physical restraints. Gerontologist 1992;32: 762–6.

69. Mion LC, Minnick A, Palmer R. Physical restraint use in the hospital setting: unresolved issues and directions for research. Milbank Q 1996;74:411–33.
70. Shorr RI, Guillen MK, Rosenblatt LC, et al. Restraint use, restraint orders, and the risk of falls in hospitalized patients. J Am Geriatr Soc 2002;50:526–9.
71. Frank C, Hodgetts G, Puxty J. Safety and efficacy of physical restraints for the elderly. Review of the evidence. Can Fam Physician 1996;42:2402–9.
72. Marks W. Physical restraints in the practice of medicine. Current concepts. Arch Intern Med 1992;152:2203–6.
73. Minnick AF, Fogg L, Mion LC, et al. Resource clusters and variation in physical restraint use. J Nurs Scholarsh 2007;39:363–70.
74. Heinze C, Dassen T, Grittner U. Use of physical restraints in nursing homes and hospitals and related factors: a cross-sectional study. J Clin Nurs 2012;21: 1033–40.
75. Centers for Medicare and Medicare Services (CMS), DHSS. 42 CFR 482. Medicare and Medicaid programs; hospital conditions of participation: patients' rights: final rule. Fed Regist 2006;71:71377–428.
76. The Joint Commission. Hospital accreditation standards (HAS) 2007. Oakbrook Terrace (IL): JCAHO; 2006.
77. Chari S, Haines T, Varghese P, et al. Are non-slip socks really 'non-slip'? An analysis of slip resistance. BMC Geriatr 2009;9:39.
78. Hartung B, Lalonde M. The use of non-slip socks to prevent falls among hospitalized older adults: a literature review. Geriatr Nurs 2017;38(5):412–6.
79. Mahida N, Boswell T. Non-slip socks: a potential reservoir for transmitting multidrug-resistant organisms in hospitals? J Hosp Infect 2016;94:273–5.
80. Haines TP, Bennell KL, Osborne RH, et al. Effectiveness of targeted falls prevention programme in subacute hospital setting: randomised controlled trial. BMJ 2004;328:676.
81. Healey F, Monro A, Cockram A, et al. Using targeted risk factor reduction to prevent falls in older in-patients: a randomised controlled trial. Age Ageing 2004;33: 390–5.
82. Cumming RG, Sherrington C, Lord SR, et al. Cluster randomised trial of a targeted multifactorial intervention to prevent falls among older people in hospital. BMJ 2008;336:758–60.
83. Barker AL, Morello RT, Wolfe R, et al. 6-PACK programme to decrease fall injuries in acute hospitals: cluster randomised controlled trial. BMJ 2016;352:h6781.
84. Cameron ID, Gillespie LD, Robertson MC, et al. Interventions for preventing falls in older people in care facilities and hospitals. Cochrane Database Syst Rev 2012;(12):CD005465. https://doi.org/10.1002/14651858.CD005465.pub4.
85. DiBardino D, Cohen ER, Didwania A. Meta-analysis: multidisciplinary fall prevention strategies in the acute care inpatient population. J Hosp Med 2012;7: 497–503.

Printed and bound by CPI Group (UK) Ltd, Croydon, CR0 4YY

03/10/2024

01040406-0014